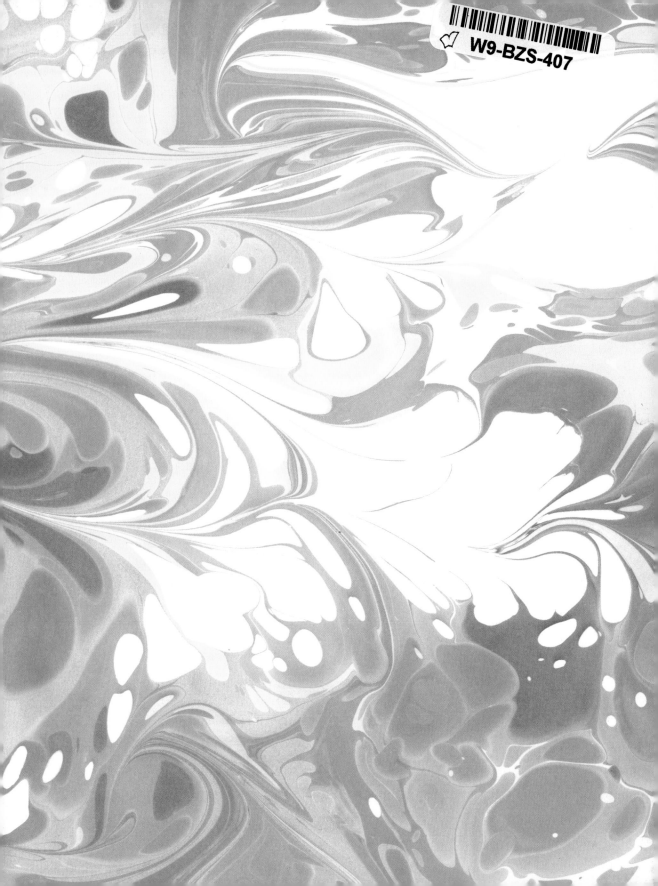

"A fresh take and clear guide to cooking with cannabis, *Edibles* is an essential makeover for infused treats. Gone are the stale pot brownies of yesteryear. In their place, Stephanie and Coreen demonstrate how to micro-dose delicious bites and pantry staples."

— VANESSA LAVORATO

Co-host of *Bong Appétit* & founder of Marigold Sweets

"If you want to learn about and understand how to cook with cannabis, Stephanie and Coreen will take you on an edible journey of creativity and technique! A must-have addition to your culinary library. Bravo!"

— MINDY SEGAL

James Beard Award-winning pastry chef, chef/owner of HotChocolate, creator of Mindy's Artisanal Edibles, and author of *Cookie Love*

EDIBLES

Dedicated to my love, for always
believing this kitchen goose could fly.

— SH

For my booski, parents, and siblings,
you are my special special humans.

— CC

Library of Congress Cataloging-in-Publication Data:
Names: Hua, Stephanie, author. | Carroll, Coreen.
Title: Edibles : Small bites for the modern cannabis kitchen / by Stephanie
  Hua ; with Coreen Carroll.
Description: San Francisco, California : Chronicle Books, LLC, [2019] |
  Includes bibliographical references and index.
Identifiers: LCCN 2018002678 (print) | LCCN 2018020546 (ebook) | ISBN
  9781452170558 | ISBN 9781452170442 (alk. paper)
Subjects: LCSH: Cooking (Marijuana) | Snack foods. | LCGFT: Cookbooks.
Classification: LCC TX819.M25 (ebook) | LCC TX819.M25 H83 2019 (print) | DDC
  641.6/379—dc23
LC record available at https://lccn.loc.gov/2018002678

Manufactured in China

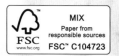

MIX
Paper from
responsible sources
FSC™ C104723
www.fsc.org

Design by Lizzie Vaughan
Marble Patterns by Shaine Drake
Typeset in TT Norms and Zahrah

Photographs by Linda Xiao
Prop Styling by Glenn Jenkins
Food Styling by Stephanie Hua and Coreen Carroll
Photographs pages 2, 136 by Stephanie Hua
Photograph page 144 by Craig Hackey

10 9 8 7 6 5

Chronicle books and gifts are available at special quantity discounts to corporations,
professional associations, literacy programs, and other organizations. For details
and discount information, please contact our corporate/premiums department at
corporatesales@chroniclebooks.com or at 1-800-759-0190.

Chronicle Books LLC
680 Second Street
San Francisco, California 94107
www.chroniclebooks.com

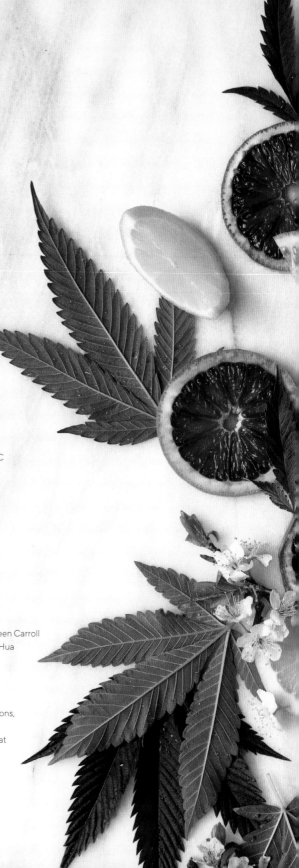

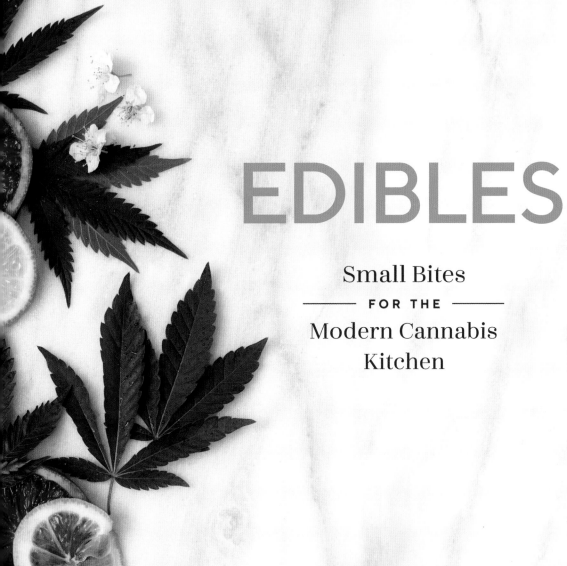

EDIBLES

Small Bites

—— FOR THE ——

Modern Cannabis Kitchen

STEPHANIE HUA

WITH COREEN CARROLL

PHOTOGRAPHS BY LINDA XIAO

CHRONICLE BOOKS

SAN FRANCISCO

Contents

OUTRO / 137

Intro

Have you ever had pot brownies from a boxed mix that tasted vaguely of burnt rubber tires and were *way* too strong (discovered, regrettably, after it was all too late)? We've been there. Let's chalk it up to being young and undiscerning. That was then, and this is now.

Pot brownies have come a long way. They can now be a gourmet experience, made from scratch with high-quality chocolate, premium cannabis, carefully infused butter, and a taste so heavenly you'll need to make a nonmedicated batch for the munchies that will—inevitably—follow.

When it comes to edibles, brownies are just the tip of the iceberg. With the end of cannabis prohibition, both the medicinal and recreational use of this magical plant is steadily normalizing. James Beard Award-winning chefs are coming out with edible lines. Talented producers are making incredible, creative goods that look right at home in a fancy boutique or the local farmers' market. Small-batch jams, jewel-like *pâte de fruits*, French macarons—even handcrafted marshmallows—have found their way into the cannabis kitchen.

Edibles are perhaps the most approachable form of consumption, and are, without a doubt, the most versatile, discreet, and delicious. If you are curious about cooking with cannabis in your own kitchen, this book teaches you how. We cover the basics about this special ingredient, explain techniques for infusion, highlight some of the industry's most innovative producers, and, of course, share our favorite recipes. These are edibles your past self could never have imagined. Edibles all grown up—gorgeous, gourmet, and carefully dosed.

FOOD + CANNABIS

Fine food and fine cannabis were meant to be together. On their own, they are super enjoyable. But together? Now that's a recipe for a good time. Used judiciously, cannabis in food can make for a complementary, enhanced experience. We also believe it is no coincidence that both bring people together. Whether you are passing a dish around the dinner table or passing a joint, you are sharing something special. You are connecting and, hopefully, laughing.

These small-bite, low-dose edibles are meant to be shared and savored. In today's hustle and bustle we believe it is important to slow down and make time for one another—and for yourself. Whether planning a hike with a friend, hosting a wake-and-bake brunch, or looking to send your dinner party guests off with a little elevated treat, these edibles will make those experiences that much more memorable.

COOKING STYLE

When we sat down to compile the recipes we wanted to share, we found ourselves with enough recipes to fill three books. Both Coreen and I are food lovers—we love to cook, and we love to feed people. We attended the same culinary school in San Francisco and our paths crossed again, years later, when we both found ourselves applying our culinary skills to cannabis. Coreen made her foray into the edibles world by making award-winning macarons (Blueberry Lemon Macarons, page 131), and now puts on incredible food and cannabis pairing events. I found myself elbow deep in rainbow sprinkles and dedicated myself to elevating the edibles experience by bringing low-dose, gourmet marshmallows (Birthday Cake Mellows, page 66) to market. The recipes you'll find in this book represent how we like to eat and entertain. We've drawn from our experience both as hosts and guests, and the resulting compilation is an all-star cast of our go-to dishes. We hope they serve you as well as they have us.

There is a range of recipes—from simple, approachable, and familiar to showstopping dishes that are more ambitious. There is also a balance between indulgent treats and healthier options. There is something for everyone!

The flavors and techniques we've created are a unique reflection of our own ever-evolving identity as curious cooks. Everything we make is influenced by our history, our food memories, our present-day environment. You'll recognize some classic favorites, remixed with a modern twist. There will be some unexpected flavor combinations, too. Trust, and roll with it!

We highlight seasonal fresh ingredients whenever possible because we think you should be gorging on candy-sweet tomatoes in summertime, and reveling in spring's first shoots of green garlic. But we also understand that's not always realistic. Good thing chocolate is always in season!

LOW DOSE, SMALL BITES

We designed our recipes to be gently dosed at approximately **5 mg THC per serving**. The small serving size makes it easy to control the dosage that's right for you.

It should be noted that 5 mg is a target, not a guarantee. Without lab testing to confirm the exact potency of your infusion, it is impossible to determine the exact potency of your finished edible. Even if you do know the potency of your infusion, there will always be a margin of variance due to cooking technique (equal distribution, equal portioning, burn off variables). This is where cooking with cannabis is closer to an art than a science. At the end of the day, our guideline will help you produce low-dose edibles that should fall within a range of **3 to 7 mg THC per serving**. Always try a small piece and see how you feel before consuming, say, half a tray of brownies (see How to Enjoy Edibles, page 15).

Low-dose edibles are meant to enhance—not impair. We often use the analogy of going into a liquor store. There are many options to choose from. You can pick up a bottle of wine, or you can grab a handle of Everclear. There's a use case for each scenario. What we're going for here is more of a rosé-all-day vibe. Let's make some tasty edibles, and let's not fuck up our friends.

Let's make some tasty edibles, and let's not fuck up our friends.

The Importance of Cannabis

Cannabis is an incredible plant that has been used throughout history, across cultures, for its unique medicinal and spiritual properties. It is insanely complex, and we're still discovering more about it each day. Let's get to know this special ingredient a little more before we get into the kitchen.

WHAT TO LOOK FOR

When you go to select your cannabis, you will be met with a dizzying array of choices. The first way to narrow your selection is by species: **sativa, indica,** or, usually, a **hybrid** of the two.

Sativas are generally known as "daytime" strains because they impart an uplifting, energetic, head high. Indicas, on the other hand, are better suited for "nighttime" enjoyment because they typically give you more of a body high, making you feel relaxed, mellow, and sometimes sleepy.

The look of the flowers even mimics these attributes. Sativa buds are tall and airy (imagine your head in the clouds), while indica buds are dense and plump (imagine sinking into a cushy couch).

Hybrids provide a combination of effects to give you the best of both worlds, leaning toward one spectrum or the other, depending on whether they are sativa dominant or indica dominant. The crossbreeding and creation of new hybrid strains give growers endless opportunities to experiment and create new strains, all of which will have their own unique set of qualities and effects.

Most dispensaries are staffed with highly knowledgeable budtenders who can help you choose a strain that's a good fit for your needs. Don't be shy about talking to them about the desired effects you're looking for.

SPOT CHECK

✓ **Strain**

Is it a sativa, indica, or hybrid? What are its characteristics? What kind of high can you expect?

✓ **Potency**

What percentage THC/CBD is it? What is its cannabinoid profile? (see Cannabinoids: Effects + Benefits, page 10).

✓ **Odor**

How does the flower smell? Aroma and flavor are inextricably connected. Seventy-five to 95 percent of what we taste is actually smell, and that absolutely applies to cannabis. If it smells good, it will probably taste good, too.

✓ **Terpene**

Terpenes are the essential oils in the plant you smell. Beyond fragrance and flavor, the distinct terpene profile of a strain also plays a role in the overall therapeutic effect. If you know which terpenes are present in the bud you are buying, you can glean a sense of how it will make you feel, or how it can help you (see Terpenes: Fragrance, Flavor + Feeling, page 11).

What to Look For

Sativa, Indica, or Hybrid?

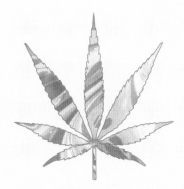

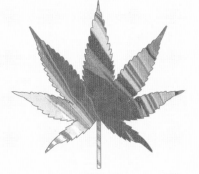

OR

SATIVA

Light color with long, thin leaves

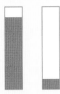

THC   CBD

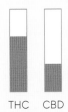

THC   CBD

INDICA

Deep color with wide, broad leaves

Airy, tall buds

Dense, plump buds

Mind | High

Creative, Euphoria, Alert,
Sociable, Cheerful, Energetic

Body | Stoned

Mellow, Sleepy, Relaxed,
Calm, Carefree, Couch lock

HYBRID

This is a crash course in how cannabis works in your body. In broad strokes, that body of yours is made up of many systems. One very important system is an internal regulatory system known as **the endocannabinoid system**. Cannabis is able to stimulate this system by introducing cannabinoids (i.e., THC, CBD), that bind to receptors in our body's cells and produce a variety of therapeutic effects. The endocannabinoid system helps regulate the nervous and immune systems via a complex group of molecules and receptors. This receptor system, thought to be the largest in the body, helps maintain many essential physiological processes including appetite, memory, blood pressure, inflammation, immunity, and pain sensation among others. Scientists believe the endocannabinoid system first evolved in primitive animals more than six hundred million years ago.

THE ENDOCANNABINOID SYSTEM HELPS REGULATE:

Bone marrow

Bones

Brain

Gastrointestinal system

Immune system

Liver

Lungs

Muscles

Pancreas

Reproductive system

Spleen

Vascular system

Both the human body and the cannabis plant produce cannabinoids that bind to receptors in the endocannabinoid system. Cannabinoids are crucial to some of the body's most basic physiological processes. To date, scientists have identified more than one hundred unique cannabinoids in cannabis (with the potential for more, since there are more than 750 distinct natural chemical components in this miracle plant that have yet to be studied in depth). Each of these chemical compounds interacts with the body's endocannabinoid system in a unique way.

Of all the cannabinoids found in cannabis, THC and CBD are the ones you'll hear about most often.

THC
THC, of course, is the most known cannabinoid, and, typically, the one found in the highest concentration. This is, in part, because for decades farmers have favored and bred high-THC plants to match the market demand. THC is *psychoactive*, which means it influences your mood and behavior. THC is responsible for the "high" feeling you get when you consume cannabis.

THC: THERAPEUTIC EFFECTS
THC has been shown to have many therapeutic benefits. It is particularly effective in mitigating pain, lack of appetite, nausea, vomiting, and muscle spasticity. It can also help relieve intraocular pressure in patients with glaucoma. Recent studies suggest that THC may be useful in managing insomnia, fatigue, PTSD, and depression.

CBD
CBD is the second-most studied plant-based cannabinoid after THC. It is *nonpsychoactive* and can even counter some of the psychoactive effects of THC. It is known for its pain-relieving and anti-inflammatory effects on the body.

CBD: THERAPEUTIC EFFECTS

Studies have suggested a wide range of CBD's possible therapeutic effects on several conditions, including Parkinson's disease, Alzheimer's disease, cerebral ischemia, diabetes, rheumatoid arthritis and other inflammatory diseases, nausea, and cancer. The reduced psychoactivity of CBD-rich cannabis may make it an appealing treatment option for patients seeking anti-inflammatory, antianxiety, antispasmodic, and/or pain-relieving effects without feeling "stoned."

While each cannabinoid works independently, when used together they interact synergistically to create what's referred to as the "entourage effect," where the therapeutic benefits of each individual component become magnified. In other words, the medicinal impact of the whole plant is greater than the sum of its parts. "Cannabis is inherently polypharmaceutical," explains leading cannabis researcher Dr. John McPartland. "Synergy arises from interactions between its multiple components." Like Captain Planet.

TERPENES: FRAGRANCE, FLAVOR + FEELING

Cannabinoids aren't the only compounds at play when it comes to determining the effects of a particular strain. Terpenes, or terpenoids, are also an important factor and play a role in the overall entourage effect. Cannabinoid-terpenoid interactions amplify the beneficial effects of cannabis while mitigating feelings of anxiety that can sometimes be brought on by THC.

What exactly are terpenes? When you take a whiff of that premium bud, that explosion of aroma that hits you in the face—those are terpenes. When you take a hit off a joint and it tastes piney or lemony—those are terpenes. And, when you feel relaxed and calm, or uplifted, after consuming cannabis, you got it—terpenes (think of it as cannabis aromatherapy).

Terpenes are the plant's essential oils. More than two hundred terpenes have been identified in the cannabis plant, and every strain of cannabis possesses its own unique terpene type and composition to give it its distinct fragrance, flavor, and feeling.

The diversity of flavors in cannabis is impressive enough, but, arguably, the most fascinating characteristic of terpenes is their ability to interact synergistically with the cannabinoids in the plant to create an entourage effect of pharmacological benefits.

Some terpenes bind to the same receptor sites as cannabinoids, affecting their chemical output. Others can modify how much THC passes through to your brain. Their hand of influence even reaches to neurotransmitters, such as dopamine and serotonin, by altering their rate of production and destruction, their movement, and the availability of receptors.

In sum, don't forget about terpenes.

The entourage effect: The whole plant is greater than its parts.

Cannabinoids

THC

Delta 9-tetrahydrocannabinol (THC) is the primary psychoactive cannabinoid in cannabis. It is responsible for the "high" effect, and much of the plant's therapeutic properties. THC is found in nine variations, with slight differences in chemical structure (for example, THCV and THCA).

CBD

Cannabidiol (CBD) is nonpsychoactive, but it has tremendous medical potential. When the correct ratio of CBD to THC is applied to treat a specific condition, it can be particularly effective. CBD also has a marked affinity for serotonin receptors, which are associated with psychological well-being.

CBN

Cannabinol (CBN) is a mildly psychoactive cannabinoid produced by the degradation of THC after it is harvested. Most fresh cannabis contains very low levels of CBN, but curing, poor storage, or processing can cause the THC content to be oxidized into CBN, creating a sedative effect known as "couch lock."

THCA

Tetrahydrocannabinolic Acid (THCA) is the most dominant compound in fresh, undried cannabis. It is the acid form of THC with a carboxyl group (-CO2H or -COOH) attached. When cannabis is burned, vaporized, or heated to a certain temperature, this carboxyl group is removed, thereby converting the THCA into THC. This activation process is called decarboxylation. Although THCA has nonpsychoactive effects, it possesses many therapeutic effects.

THCV

Tetrahydrocannabivarin (THCV) is a variant of THC. It is believed to be an appetite suppressant, and can have sedative effects, making it useful for the reduction of panic attacks. Although THCV's psychoactivity appears to be less than THC, it is usually associated with extremely potent cannabis.

CBG

Cannabigerol (CBG) is a nonpsychoactive cannabinoid that is the parent cannabinoid to THC and CBD. Not all strains contain CBG, but, in the ones that do, the CBG starts to convert to THC and CBD as the plant matures. To capture it, the flower must be harvested during the early stages of flowering.

CBC

Cannabichromene (CBC) is potentially one of the most important cannabinoids. Cells responsible for memory and learning are continuously made via a process called neurogenesis, and CBC is found to increase the viability of those cells.

CBDA

Cannabidiolic Acid (CBDA) is a nonpsychoactive cannabinoid believed to have anti-inflammatory properties. Similar to THCA, CBDA can be converted to CBD through decarboxylation. The largest quantities of CBDA are found in the raw (unheated, uncured) flowers of CBD-rich plants.

CBDV

Cannabidivarin (CBDV) is a close relative of CBD. Studies have shown promise for its use in treating epilepsy.

Therapeutic Effects

Psychiatric & Neurological Disorders

Anti-anxiety	CBD
Antidepressant	CBD, **THC**
Antiepileptic	CBD, THCV
Antipsychotic	CBD
Antispasmodic	CBD, **CBN**, **THC**, THCA
Neuroprotective	CBD

Eating & Digestive Disorders

Aids digestion	CBD, **CBDA**
Antibacterial	CBD, **CBG**
Antimicrobial	CBC
Antinausea	CBD, **THC**
Antioxidant	**CBN**, **THC**
Appetite stimulant	THC
Appetite suppressant	THCV

Pain & Sleep Issues

Aids sleep	CBN
Anti-inflammatory	CBC, CBD, **CBG**, **CBN**, THCA
Anti-sleep apnea	THC
Relieves pain	CBC, CBD, **CBN**, THC

Specific Diseases & Other Benefits

Aids artery blockage	CBD
Aids blood flow	CBD
Aids bone growth	CBC, CBD, CBDV, **CBG**, THCV
Aids psoriasis	CBD
Allograft stimulant (minimizes organ rejection)	CBD
Antidiabetic	CBD
Immunosuppressive	CBD
Inhibits tumor cell growth	CBC, CBD, **CBDA**, **CBG**, THCA
Reduces pressure from glaucoma	THC
Restricts blood flow	CBC

Terpenes

Fragrance, Flavor, and Feeling

MYRCENE

Aromas/Flavors: cloves, earthy musk, tropical fruit

Therapeutic Effects: antidepressant, sedative, muscle relaxant, pain relief, anti-inflammatory

Also Found In: hops, mango, lemongrass, pineapple

CARYOPHYLLENE

Aromas/Flavors: cedar, oregano, black pepper

Therapeutic Effects: neuroprotective, anticancer, anti-inflammatory, gastroprotective

Also Found In: cinnamon, black pepper, echinacea, Thai basil

LIMONENE

Aromas/Flavors: citrus, juniper, peppermint

Therapeutic Effects: anti-anxiety, antidepressant, gastroprotective

Also Found In: juniper, lemons, peppermint

HUMULENE

Aromas/Flavors: earth, funk, wood

Therapeutic Effects: pain relief, anti-inflammatory, suppresses appetite

Also Found In: beer, cheese

LINALOOL

Aromas/Flavors: citrus, flowers

Therapeutic Effects: sedative, anti-anxiety, anticonvulsant

Also Found In: basil, lavender, mint

NEROLIDOL

Aromas/Flavors: berries, flowers, pine

Therapeutic Effects: antifungal, sedative, skin protectant

Also Found In: ginger, jasmine, lemongrass, orange peel

PINENE

Aromas/Flavors: pine, rosemary

Therapeutic Effects: antibacterial, aids breathing, aids memory, anti-inflammatory

Also Found In: basil, dill, parsley, pine needles

Cooking with Cannabis

Now that you have a more complete
appreciation of how magical cannabis is, let's
get to the fun stuff—cooking and eating it!

4 STEPS TO MAKING EDIBLES:

1. Calculate Dosage

2. Decarboxylate

3. Make an Infusion

4. Find a Recipe

INGESTING CANNABIS

First, we should point out, ingesting cannabis is an entirely different ballgame from smoking it. There are a few main points to note.

LONGER ONSET

When you smoke or vape cannabis, you can feel the effects within minutes. Because of the way ingested cannabis is metabolized, the effect of edibles can take anywhere from 30 minutes to 2 hours to hit—in some cases even longer. Because you can't feel the effects right away when you ingest cannabis, it can be easy to overdo. As you embark on your edibles journey, a good rule of thumb is start low, go slow.

LONGER LASTING

The high you experience from smoked cannabis usually lasts from 1 to 3 hours. Ingested cannabis produces a longer-lasting high that can last from 3 to 7 hours, sometimes more depending on the dose.

MORE INTENSE

When you smoke cannabis, THC is absorbed through your lungs and travels to your brain to get you high. When you ingest cannabis, that same THC travels through the stomach and is metabolized in the liver, which then allows it to cross the blood-brain barrier more effectively, resulting in a more intense high.

HOW TO ENJOY EDIBLES

When experimenting with edibles, start with a small amount, wait up to 2 hours to gauge its effect, then decide if you want to eat more. Edibles are notoriously difficult to dose consistently— even with professionally packaged edibles, you can have two different products, both touting the same dosage, that feel very different. If you want to be cautious, it's not a bad idea to repeat this exercise each time you try a new batch of edibles.

Everyone reacts differently to ingested cannabis. Your body weight and metabolism play a part, as does your tolerance level (smoking tolerance, by the way, is different from edibles tolerance), and variables such as whether you consume it on an empty stomach.

If you have never experimented with edibles before, we recommend starting with a **1- to 5-mg THC dose**. If you occasionally dabble, or have a moderate tolerance, you may prefer a dose of **5 to 10 mg of THC**. Once you learn how edibles affect you, you can set and adjust your dose as needed to ensure a safe and enjoyable experience.

If you've overdone it, relax, breathe, and rest assured knowing no one has ever died from a cannabis overdose. (Opioid overdoses, on the other hand, take an estimated 69,000 lives each year worldwide, according to the World Health Organization . . . We'll just leave that fact right here.)

DOSAGE

The recipes in this book have been developed with a target dose of approximately **5 mg THC per serving**. Following our guidelines, your edibles should fall within a range of **3 to 7 mg THC per serving**. This is considered a low, or micro, dose. In our experience, doses within this range are approachable and easy to control and adjust until you find your sweet spot.

Remember, the effect of an edible can take up to 2 hours to hit, so wait before ingesting more. You can always eat more; you can never eat less. Start low, go slow, and find the dose that works for you.

If you are new to edibles, have a lower tolerance, or simply prefer a more mellow experience, we recommend following our dosage as written in the recipes.

If you'd like to increase the potency of the recipe, you can adjust the amount of infusion in most of the recipes as long as you keep the ratios in balance. For example, if a recipe calls for 3 Tbsp [42 g] unsalted butter and 1 Tbsp [13 g] canna butter, and you'd like to double the strength of the recipe, adjust the quantities to 2 Tbsp [28 g] unsalted butter and 2 Tbsp [26 g] canna butter. Or just eat double the amount!

INFUSION POTENCY

Infusion potency is dependent on the potency of your cannabis to start, prior to decarbing. Every strain varies in its percentage of THC; in fact, even different harvests of the same strain can vary in potency depending on growing condition variables and curing time, so it's best practice to know what you're starting with.

When you obtain your cannabis, make note of its combined THC + THCA percentage. **If you are working with a strain that is approximately 23 percent combined THC + THCA, your master infusions should yield comparable potencies.**

It is important to note that the only way to truly know the strength of your infusion is to have it lab tested. Many labs offer discounted testing to individuals looking to test for personal use (see Resources, page 137). There are also home tools that can measure the potency of oil, butter, or tincture infusions (see Resources, page 137).

Start low, go slow, and find the dose that works for you.

Dosage Calculation

Our recipes were developed using Sour Diesel flower that measured

1.39% THC & 21.74% THCA

Using this flower, our master infusions yielded the following potencies:

INFUSION	POTENCY (MG THC/G)	POTENCY (MG THC/TSP)
Canna Butter (page 27)	7.53	32.38
Canna Coconut Oil (page 29)	6.27	26.96
Canna Tincture (page 33)	10.04	40.16
Canna Honey (page 34)	0.82	5
Canna Maple Syrup (page 35)	0.91	5

Test results provided by CW Analytical. For more information, see Resources, page 137.

Then we calculated the amount of infusion needed for each recipe:

Desired Dosage per Serving (mg THC)	X	Number of Servings in Recipe		Infusion Potency (mg THC/g)	=	Amount of Infusion Needed for Recipe (g)

For recipes that require baking or heating, we increase the amount of infusion used to adjust for burn-off loss (typically by about 13 percent).

For example, if you want to make a batch of 12 cookies that are 5 mg THC per cookie, using canna butter that is 7.53 mg THC/gram in potency, the calculation would be: 5 x 12 ÷ 7.53 = 7.97 grams of canna butter needed for your recipe.

Tricks of the Trade

As you've probably noticed by now, cannabis cooking is unlike other types of cooking. There is a level of precision to consider, especially when working with low-dose edibles. Here are some tricks we've learned along the way that can make navigating this brave new world a little easier.

TOOLS FOR THE MODERN CANNABIS KITCHEN

Digital scale

Stand mixer

Food processor

Instant-read or candy thermometer

Flexible rubber spatulas

Pastry scraper

Fine-mesh strainer

Cheesecloth

Silicone mats or parchment paper

Baking pans, sheets, and saucepans

Cookie scoops

Pastry bags and decorative tips

Coffee grinder or spice grinder

Latex or rubber gloves

Shot glass

Glass jars with lids

Offset spatula

Sous vide machine

TIPS + TECHNIQUES

Cook smarter, not harder. We've figured these out so you don't have to. Use the following tips for better results every time.

CONSISTENCY IS KEY

Whether we're talking about consistent mixing (scrape down the sides of your mixer bowl and, while you're at it, get into that little divot at the bottom of the bowl where the whisk can never reach), equal distribution of batter in a pan, or equal portioning, always have the goal of consistency in mind.

WEIGH YOUR INGREDIENTS AND PORTIONS

We feel truly, madly, deeply about this—weigh your cannabis, weigh all your ingredients, weigh out your portions. A good digital scale will change how you cook, with cannabis or otherwise, but particularly when working with an ingredient such as cannabis where the difference of a few grams can matter. It is the most accurate way to make sure each serving gets the same amount of medicated goodness. We do provide options, like using Tbsp measures or cookie scoops, to portion without a scale. But really, please use a scale. We promise your results will be better.

LEVEL YOUR SCOOP AND SPOON MEASURES

Begin by taking a heaping mound of the ingredient. Allow it to overflow. Using the flat edge of a pastry scraper or the back of a knife, tap the edge of the scoop to help make sure it is completely filled, and slide it across the edge of the scoop to give you a consistent measurement each time. If you're scooping something sticky, like dough, scrape out all the dough from the scoop each time.

LIMIT HEAT EXPOSURE WHENEVER POSSIBLE
Always be aware of how much heat you expose your infusions to and limit that exposure as much as possible. Excessive heat can quickly burn off precious THC and other cannabinoids. Our recipes have been adjusted to account for heat loss where applicable. As a general rule of thumb, we try not to let the internal temperature of an edible exceed 350°F [180°C].

USE A RUBBER SPATULA
There are many uses for a rubber spatula, but the most important one—when it comes to cannabis cooking—is to make sure you're not wasting any medicated goods by leaving them behind in a bowl or pan. Scrape it all out and be thorough!

SOFTENING BUTTER
If you happen to make a recipe on a whim and don't have time to let your butter naturally come to room temperature, here's a favorite hack for getting it soft STAT: Place the cold butter on a plate. Fill a large liquid measuring cup or glass bowl with boiling water and let it sit for 1 to 2 minutes. Empty the water and dry the container. Quickly place it over the butter, creating a little steam sauna. Let it sit for a few minutes while you prep your recipe. By the time you're ready, your butter will be nice and relaxed!

LINING A BAKING PAN
Spray the pan with nonstick baking spray and line it with parchment paper, leaving an overhang of 2 in [5 cm] on each side. Fold the overhang in on each side until it neatly fits into the bottom of the pan. Lift the flaps, creasing the paper at the corners so it is flush against the pan and doesn't bunch up. This ensures your batter gets into the corners evenly. That makes the consistency gods happy.

MAKING A DOUBLE BOILER
A double boiler is our go-to method for melting chocolate because the gentle heat from the steam melts the chocolate evenly and slowly, without risk of burning it. To make a double boiler, simply fill a medium saucepan with 1 to 2 in [3 to 5 cm] of water and bring to barely a simmer over medium-high heat. Adjust the heat to low. Place whatever you're melting in a heatproof bowl (stainless steel or tempered glass) over the saucepan. The bowl should be big enough so that the bottom of the bowl does not touch the water. Stir the contents occasionally with a rubber spatula. Once your ingredient is melted, remove the bowl from the heat. Wipe the bottom of the bowl with a kitchen towel to prevent water splashing onto your work surface. Alternatively, if you want to use the microwave, microwave your ingredient using short bursts (15 to 30 seconds at a time) and stir in between to ensure your chocolate doesn't burn.

WORK CLEANLY AND EFFICIENTLY
Something we've learned working in professional kitchens is the value of working cleanly and efficiently. Before you do anything, read the recipe in its entirety so there are no surprises in the middle of cooking. Set up your *mise en place* (French for "everything in its place")—organize and measure your ingredients, assemble the equipment you need, and get everything ready. This way you can work efficiently through the recipe without having to stop for each ingredient. Failing to plan is planning for failure. Oh, and always clean as you go.

CLEARLY LABEL AND DATE ALL INFUSIONS AND EDIBLES FOR STORAGE
The last thing you want is Grandma finding your stash of medicated caramels in the freezer and

putting them out for her knitting group. Including the date is a good idea to make sure you consume the foods while they're still good.

WORKING WITH A PASTRY BAG AND TIP

Disposable plastic pastry bags are the best. You can hack one out of a resealable plastic bag as well. Cut off the tip. Insert the decorative tip you plan to use into the bag to gauge how much you'll need to cut off for it to fit. Do not cut off too much or your piping tip may slip out while you are piping your mixture. Slip the tip into the bag and place it snugly into the small opening. Place the bag in a tall glass or deli container and fold the top over to form a cuff over the rim. You now have both hands free to fill the bag. Fill your bag using a rubber spatula for easy scraping.

Once the filling has been added, push all the mixture toward the tip of the bag, allowing any air to escape. Twist the top of the bag shut to prevent any mixture from spilling out. With your dominant hand, hold the piping bag toward the top (at the twist), not at the bottom. If this feels awkward, try filling the bag less full so you have more control. Use your opposite hand to guide the bag and hold it steady as you pipe. While piping don't press the tip directly against the surface, as this does not give the filling anywhere to go. Rather, hold it just off the surface at a constant height as you pipe.

Apply pressure to the bag by slowly closing your dominant hand (the one at the top of the bag) until the filling begins to flow out. Pipe slowly and steadily. As you reach the desired size, stop squeezing, and make a quick flicking motion, like the shape of a comma, as you lift the tip. Reposition and pipe the next shape. As you pipe, twist the top of the bag closed. This helps push your mixture out of the bag evenly. Continue piping, refilling the bag as needed.

MACARON PIPING MADE EASY

A great way to help you pipe consistent circles is using a guide. On a piece of parchment paper measured to fit your baking sheet and using a 1½-in [4 cm] round cookie cutter, trace twenty circles (four rows of five) about 1½ in [4 cm] apart, staggering the rows. Flip the parchment over, ink-side down, and you're ready to pipe. Alternatively, you can print a "macaron stencil" guideline from the Internet. Place it beneath your parchment paper or silicone baking mat (you'll be able to see the circles through the parchment when it's time to pipe). Remove the stencil before baking.

ENTERTAINING TIPS

At the heart of this book about food and cannabis is the concept of community. Nothing brings people together like food and weed. Imagine bringing together your favorite people to enjoy the fruits of your labor. They will be so impressed! We hope the recipes that follow find a way to your table and play a small part in creating some great memories.

Whether an intimate dinner party or high tea for a group, there's nothing we love more than throwing a good party. Here are some tips we've learned along the way:

- Welcome guests with a low-dose mocktail—the Peach & Ginger Ale Float (page 41) will knock their socks off. This sets the carefree tone as soon as they arrive. Avoid serving too much alcohol as it can intensify and change the true effects of the cannabis.

- Education is key when throwing your own infused party. Make sure people are aware of how strong everything is, what they should expect (see Ingesting Cannabis, page 15), and how they should properly dose themselves (see How to Enjoy Edibles, page 15). As a host, there is nothing worse than sending your guests into a bad trip, so make sure everyone is educated before they dig in.

- Have lots and lots of water available. Spa water is easy and fun—just add lemon slices and fresh mint to a pitcher of ice water. If you want to go the extra mile, a nonalcoholic option in an unexpected flavor is a nice touch (think elderflower lemonade or ginger-hibiscus iced tea).

- Good music, good lighting, and a little decor are elements of any great party, canna or otherwise. Have a few playlists ready to match the ebb and flow of the party's energy level, string some twinkle lights if you're outside, or set the table with a few touches of greenery. If you have access to them, cannabis leaves make a great addition to flower arrangements or other table decor. Set the tone and make people feel comfortable.

- Low-dose small bites lend themselves perfectly for entertaining. People will want to try everything. Give them the option of trying various infused bites, but keep them low-dosed enough so they can graze without overdoing it.

- Think of cannabis as a spice. You don't want to overspice your food; you want to season it with intention. If you are using your infusions in your own recipes, experiment with flavors that complement and balance the cannabis profile.

- If you are leaving a plate of medicated food out for self-serving, or passing appetizers, clearly label the foods so no one consumes by accident.

- Anticipate munchies and always offer noninfused options to give guests a break.

- The CBD cannabinoid can help mitigate the psychoactive effects of THC, so we like to have some on hand in case someone gets too high. You can infuse water or a nonalcoholic drink with CBD tincture, or have a few high-CBD joints ready.

- Speaking of joints, we like to pre-roll some (mark them with the strain they contain) or have vaporizers ready for those who prefer to smoke their cannabis rather than eat it. When we do flower pairings at a meal, we serve a sativa-dominant strain at the beginning to amplify the energy and excitement of the party, CBD gets introduced in the middle when guests are at peak euphoria, and we wind things down with an indica-dominant strain at the end of the meal. Have fun! Curate a selection of your favorite strains with your favorite foods and let the magic happen.

- Make sure guests get home safely. Organize car services or ask guests to plan ahead for a safe ride home through public transportation, taxi, or a designated driver.

- Everyone loves a goodie bag. Send guests home with a sample of your newfound passion. They will wake up the next morning with a tasty little treat to remind them of how much fun they had.

Think of cannabis as a spice; season with intention.

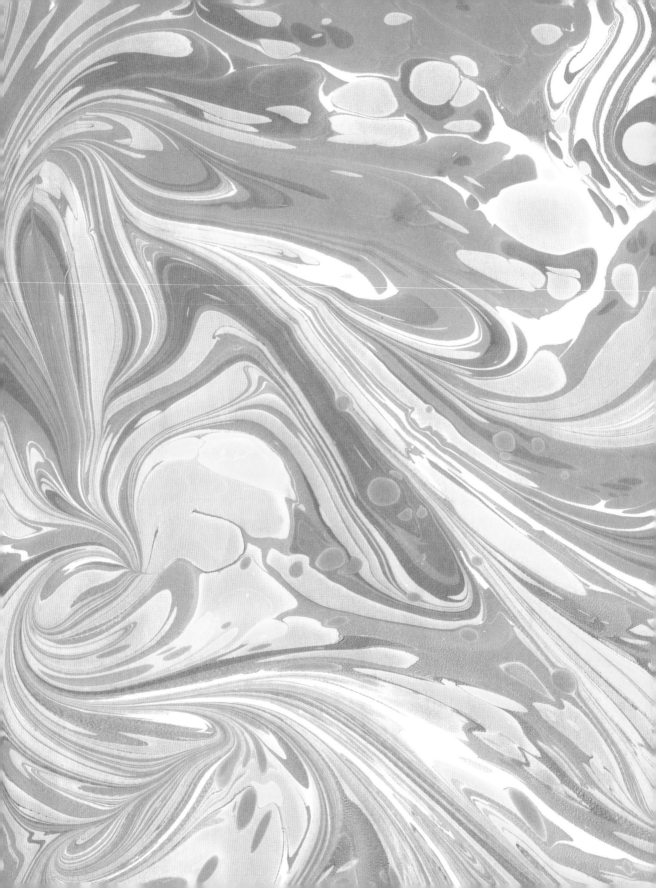

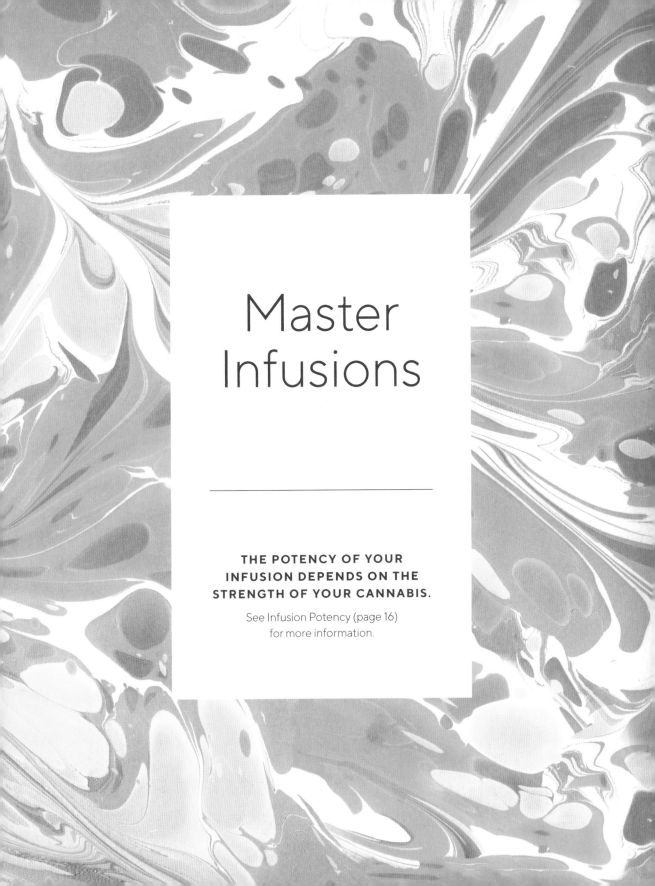

Master Infusions

THE POTENCY OF YOUR INFUSION DEPENDS ON THE STRENGTH OF YOUR CANNABIS.

See Infusion Potency (page 16) for more information.

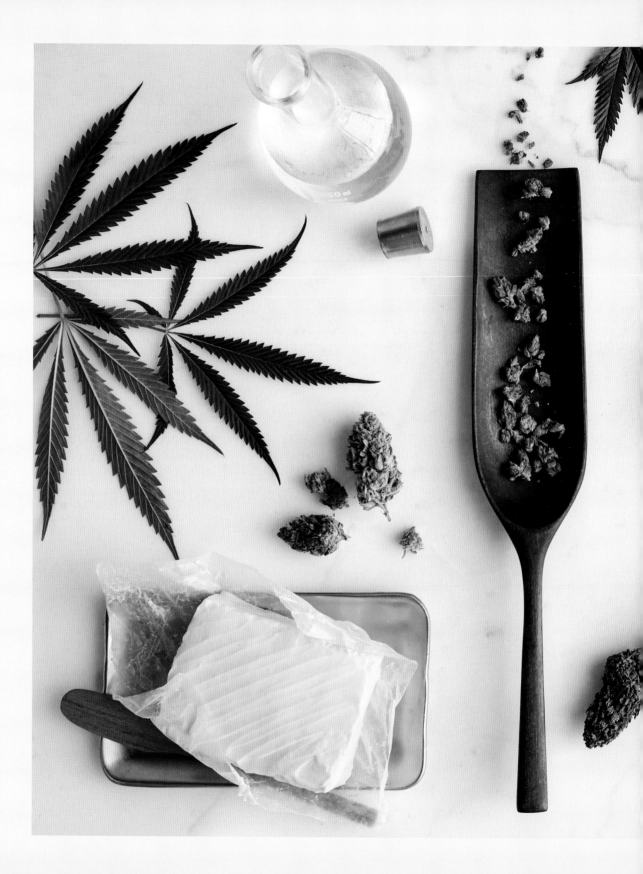

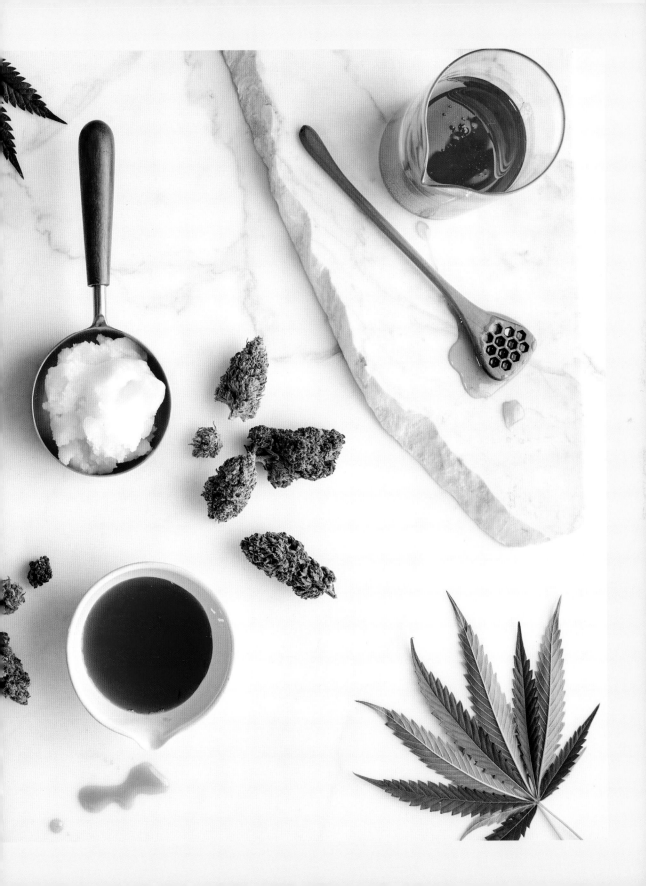

Decarboxylation: How to Activate THC

This makes the active ingredient for your Master Infusions (page 27–35).

ACTIVE TIME: **10 minutes** | INACTIVE TIME: **1 hour, 20 minutes**

We like to think of cannabis as a prized ingredient, a delicacy like a rare truffle or luxurious saffron threads. In the right hands, it can transform a dish into something transcendent. Once you unlock the mystery of working with this herb, the possibilities are limitless.

Proper decarboxylation is the key. Decarboxylation (commonly referred to as "decarbing") is the heating process in which THCA, the nonpsychoactive acid form of THC, is converted into the psychoactive cannabinoid, THC. Without this step your edibles cannot reach their full potential (i.e., they just won't get you high). So how do you do it?

1. Start with premium cannabis flower, more commonly referred to as bud. Like anything else, the better quality ingredient you start with, the better quality your end product will be—in this case, that includes taste, the potency of your infusion, and the quality of your high. We recommend weighing out a little more than you need for your infusion to account for loss in water weight during cooking. Or, if you plan on making multiple infusions, decarb all the flower you'll need at one time. This technique can be used for any amount of cannabis, as long as it fits on the pan in one even layer.

2. Preheat the oven to 275°F [135°C]. It's important to allow 1 hour for your oven to preheat to ensure the temperature is consistent throughout. Line a sheet pan with parchment paper.

3. Using scissors, snip off any large stems. With a sharp knife, chop the cannabis into small, even pea-size pieces.

4. Spread the herb evenly in a single layer on the prepared sheet pan. Bake, uninterrupted, for 20 minutes—no opening the door to peek!

5. Remove the pan from the oven and place it on a cooling rack. Once the decarbed flower is completely cooled, store it in an airtight container in the freezer until you're ready to make your infusions. The flower loses its potency over time with extended storage, so it's best to use it as soon as possible.

Note: Cooking with cannabis creates quite the aroma. If this is an issue, using a contained decarboxylation machine or a sous vide machine (see Resources, page 137) can be a good alternative.

Canna Butter

ACTIVE TIME: **30 minutes**	INACTIVE TIME: **28 hours**	MAKES: **1 cup** | **206 g**

¼ oz | 7 g decarboxylated cannabis flower

12 oz | 340 g cold unsalted butter (see Note)

2 cups | 473 g cold water

SPECIAL EQUIPMENT

Candy thermometer (optional)

Fine-mesh strainer

Cheesecloth

Tall 1-qt [960-ml] deli container or measuring cup

½-pt [240-ml] glass Mason jar with tight-fitting lid

NOTE

For our recipe we use standard American butter, which typically clocks in at around 80 percent butterfat. European-style butter will have upwards of 82 percent butterfat, which may give you a higher potency than what we've tested.

A basic building block for cooking with cannabis, canna butter is one of the most commonly used forms of infusion. Once you master this recipe, you can turn almost anything into an edible. Whether it's baked goods (Booty Call Brownies, page 76), confections (Cardamom Caramels, page 73), or savory bites (Fried Mac & Cheese Bites, page 111), use your versatile canna butter to make them extra special. For a simple transformation, stir some melted canna butter into any store-bought or homemade sauce or spread (as in the Spiced Plum Chutney component of the Duck Meatball Sliders, page 95, and our favorite Chocolate Hazelnut Spread, page 42).

In a medium saucepan over medium heat, combine the cannabis, butter, and water. Bring to just below boiling, 200°F to 210°F [95°C to 99°C], without stirring. We recommend using a candy thermometer for precision. Adjust the heat to low. Keep the mixture at this temperature for 4 hours. Using a rubber spatula, scrape down the sides of the pan if you start to see bits of herb sticking to it. The liquid will be at a constant gentle simmer. A few bubbles will break through the fat layer, but the mixture should never come to a rolling boil. If you notice the water getting low from evaporation, add 1 cup [237 g] hot tap water to prevent the mixture from burning.

After 4 hours, remove the pan from heat and let cool for 10 minutes.

CONT'D

Place a fine-mesh strainer over a large bowl and line the strainer with cheesecloth. Carefully pour in the cannabis-butter mixture. Use a rubber spatula to scrape out the pot, making sure you get all the butter and herb particles. With the spatula or the back of a ladle, press the mixture against the strainer to squeeze out all the liquid you can. Gather up the cheesecloth and give it another good press against the sieve to make sure you get out as much liquid as possible. Discard the leftover debris. (If you are making a larger batch, you may find it helpful to use a potato ricer to efficiently compress the cheesecloth-wrapped herb.)

Pour the butter-water liquid into a tall container—make sure the container isn't too wide or your butter block will be too thin and difficult to remove. Use a rubber spatula to clean the bowl; make sure you get every last bit—that's liquid gold in there! Cover and refrigerate for 24 hours.

Once the mixture cools, the butter and water will separate. Remove the butter block from the container and pat dry with a paper towel. You may have to cut around the edges or lightly push down on the sides to loosen it. If your block breaks while pulling it out, don't worry. Just make sure to get all the butter pieces out. Use a small strainer to scoop up any remaining butter bits.

On the bottom of the butter block you will see a green film. Using the back of a knife, scrape off this film and toss it along with the remaining water down the drain (see Tip).

In a small pot over low heat, melt the canna butter. Once melted, immediately turn off the heat and pour the butter into the glass jar and seal the lid. Label the jar with the date and contents. Refrigerate for up to one month, or freeze for up to six months.

Canna Coconut Oil

| ACTIVE TIME: **30 minutes** | INACTIVE TIME: **28 hours** | MAKES: **1½ cups** \| **310 g** |

¼ oz | 7 g decarboxylated cannabis flower

12 oz | 340 g coconut oil

2 cups | 473 g cold water

SPECIAL EQUIPMENT

Candy thermometer (optional)

Fine-mesh strainer

Cheesecloth

Tall 1-qt [960-ml] deli container or measuring cup

1-pt [473-ml] glass Mason jar with tight-fitting lid

Using this infusion method, you can make a number of different oils (see Variation, page 30). We chose coconut oil because of its unique properties—versatility in liquid to solid form, health benefits, high smoking point, and a high saturated fat structure that efficiently binds to ingested cannabinoids and increases their bioavailability. We also enjoy the flavor of canna coconut oil (case in point: delightful Birthday Cake Mellows, page 66; healthy Carrot Cake Energy Bites, page 46; and savory Green Eggs & Ham, page 51).

In a medium saucepan over medium heat, combine the cannabis, coconut oil, and water. Bring to just below boiling, 200°F to 210°F [95°C to 99°C], without stirring. We recommend using a candy thermometer for precision. Adjust the heat to low. Keep the mixture at this temperature for 4 hours. Using a rubber spatula, scrape down the sides of the pan if you start to see bits of herb sticking to it. The liquid will be at a constant gentle simmer. A few bubbles will break through the fat layer, but the mixture should never come to a rolling boil. If you notice the water getting low from evaporation, add 1 cup [237 g] hot tap water to prevent the mixture from burning.

After 4 hours, remove the pan from heat and let cool for 10 minutes.

Place a fine-mesh strainer over a large bowl and line the strainer with cheesecloth. Carefully pour in the cannabis-oil mixture. Use a rubber spatula to scrape out the pot, making sure you get all the oil and herb particles. With the spatula or the back of a ladle, press the mixture against the strainer to squeeze out all the liquid you can. Gather up the cheesecloth and give it another good press against the sieve to make sure you get out as much liquid as possible.

CONT'D

VARIATION

Use this recipe with other oils that solidify in the refrigerator. When making canna oils we recommend using oils with a high smoking point (avocado oil, grapeseed oil, peanut oil, canola oil, or vegetable oil). Oils with lower smoking points (olive oil, sesame oil, walnut oil, almond oil) can often taste bitter and burnt using this infusion method. For these more delicate oils, we recommend the sous vide method of infusion (see facing page). Note the recipes in this book that call for Canna Coconut Oil have been tested and dosed specifically using this infusion. Substituting another type of oil infusion in our recipes may not give you the same dosage because different oils absorb cannabis at different levels.

Discard the leftover debris. (If you are making a larger batch, you may find it helpful to use a potato ricer to efficiently compress the cheesecloth-wrapped herb.)

Pour the oil-water liquid into a tall container—make sure the container isn't too wide or your oil block will be too thin and difficult to remove. Use a rubber spatula to clean the bowl; make sure you get every last bit—that's liquid gold in there! Cover and refrigerate for 24 hours.

Once the mixture cools, the oil and water will separate. Remove the oil block from the container and pat dry with a paper towel. You may have to cut around the edges or lightly push down on the sides to loosen it. If your block breaks while pulling it out, don't worry. Just make sure to get all the solid oil pieces out. Use a small strainer to scoop up any remaining oil bits.

In a small pot over low heat, melt the canna oil. Once melted, immediately turn off the heat and pour the oil into the glass jar and seal the lid. Label the jar with the date and contents. Refrigerate for up to three months, or freeze for up to six months.

Sous Vide Canna Infusions

ACTIVE TIME: **10 minutes**	INACTIVE TIME: **4 hours**	MAKES: **¾ cup** | **155 g**

¼ oz | 7 g decarboxylated cannabis flower

6 oz | 170 g unsalted butter, melted (see Note, page 27) or coconut oil, melted

SPECIAL EQUIPMENT
Sous vide machine

½-pt [240-ml] glass Mason jar with tight-fitting lid

Fine-mesh strainer

Cheesecloth

Sous vide, which means "under vacuum" in French, is a method of cooking vacuum-sealed food in a temperature-controlled water bath heated by an immersion circulator. Professional chefs have long valued this technique for its precision and ability to produce consistent results, characteristics that make sous vide perfect for making cannabis infusions. Home sous vide machines have grown in popularity over the past few years and are widely available for the modern home cook (see Resources, page 137). Sous vide canna infusions don't require any babysitting since the temperature is automatically regulated. Added bonus: because everything is sealed, there is no smell!

Set your sous vide water bath to 185°F [85°C].

In the glass jar, combine the cannabis and melted butter or coconut oil. Secure the lid tightly and give it a good shake.

Once the machine is at temperature, place the jar in the water bath. It should be fully submerged. Process for 4 hours.

CONT'D

Transfer the jar to a counter and let cool for 5 minutes. Place a fine-mesh strainer over a medium bowl and line the strainer with cheesecloth. Pour in the cannabis-butter (or oil) mixture. Using a rubber spatula, scrape out the jar, making sure you get all the butter (or oil) and herb particles. With the spatula or the back of a spoon, press the mixture against the strainer to squeeze out all the liquid you can. Gather up the cheesecloth and give it another good press against the sieve to make sure you get out as much liquid as possible. Discard the leftover debris.

Wash and dry the glass jar and transfer the finished butter (or oil) back into it. Label the jar with the date and contents. Refrigerate to cool, and keep refrigerated for up to one month, or freeze for up to six months.

Canna Tincture

| ACTIVE TIME: **10 minutes** | INACTIVE TIME: **1 week** | MAKES: **¾ cup** \| **144 g** |

¼ oz | 7 g decarboxylated cannabis flower

¾ cup | 158 g 151-proof Everclear or pure grain alcohol

SPECIAL EQUIPMENT
½-pt [240-ml] glass Mason jar with tight-fitting lid

Fine-mesh strainer

Cheesecloth

½-pt [240-ml] dark glass jar with tight-fitting lid

Unlike canna butter or canna oil, this infusion is alcohol based rather than fat based, providing a great way to infuse edibles when the addition of butter or oil is not desired. We use this canna tincture to make our Grapefruit Negroni *"Pot" de Fruits* (page 79) jelly candies. It is also well suited for infusing beverages, as in the refreshing Peach & Ginger Ale Float (page 41). Another benefit of tinctures is that they retain a fuller spectrum of the plant's medicinal compounds because no heat is applied during the extraction process.

In the glass Mason jar, combine the cannabis and alcohol. Give it a good stir. Secure the lid tightly and place it in the freezer. Freezing means less chlorophyll will leach into your tincture, and you'll end up with a cleaner-tasting tincture.

Once a day for one week, shake the jar to mix the contents. After exactly one week, remove the jar from the freezer. Place a fine-mesh strainer over a small bowl and line the strainer with cheesecloth. Pour in the tincture mixture. Using a rubber spatula, scrape out the jar, making sure you get all the tincture and herb particles. With the spatula or the back of a spoon, press the mixture against the strainer, squeezing out all the alcohol. Gather up the cheesecloth and give it another good press against the sieve to make sure you get out as much liquid as possible. Discard the leftover debris.

Transfer the strained tincture to a dark glass jar—the darker the better because it prevents outside light from aging and degrading the herbal contents. Label the jar with the date and contents and freeze, or store in a dark cool place, for up to one year.

Canna Honey

ACTIVE TIME: **5 minutes**	INACTIVE TIME: **2 hours inactive**	MAKES: **1 cup** | **311 g**

Sweet and luscious, canna honey is a luxurious and convenient way to incorporate cannabis into your diet. We use it to medicate our superfood-charged Apple Power Crumble (page 60) and crowd-pleasing PB & J Chocolate Cups (page 115), but you could just as easily drizzle it over your morning yogurt or stir a spoonful into a cup of hot tea.

¾ cup plus 1 scant Tbsp | 273 g high-quality honey

3 Tbsp | 38 g Canna Coconut Oil (page 29), melted

SPECIAL EQUIPMENT
½-pt [240-ml] glass Mason jar with tight-fitting lid

In a blender, combine the honey and **canna coconut oil**. Blend for 1 minute on high speed until thoroughly combined and transfer to a small bowl. Using a rubber spatula, scrape down the sides of the blender to get out as much honey as possible. Place the bowl in the refrigerator for about 2 hours until the mixture is chilled.

Remove from the refrigerator and whisk the mixture thoroughly. This second mixing helps set the emulsion, making sure it is evenly blended. Transfer the honey infusion to the glass jar and secure the lid tightly. Label the jar with the date and contents. Refrigerate for up to three months.

Canna Maple Syrup

ACTIVE TIME: **5 minutes**	INACTIVE TIME: **0 minutes**	MAKES: **1 cup** | **299 g**

¾ cup plus 1 Tbsp | 261 g
Grade A maple syrup

3 Tbsp | 38 g Canna Coconut
Oil (page 29), melted

SPECIAL EQUIPMENT
½-pt [240-ml] glass Mason jar
with tight-fitting lid

If you needed a reason to make pancakes today, look no further. This canna maple syrup is tasty, easy to dose, and can be used to sweeten anything from beverages and salad dressings to the stunning Coconut Yogurt & Honeycomb (page 69). Added bonus: it's vegan friendly.

In a blender, combine the maple syrup and **canna coconut oil**. Blend for 1 minute on high speed until thoroughly combined. Transfer the syrup mixture to the glass jar. Using a rubber spatula, scrape down the sides of the blender to get out as much maple syrup as possible. Secure the lid tightly, and label the jar with the date and contents. Refrigerate for up to three months. Shake well before each use.

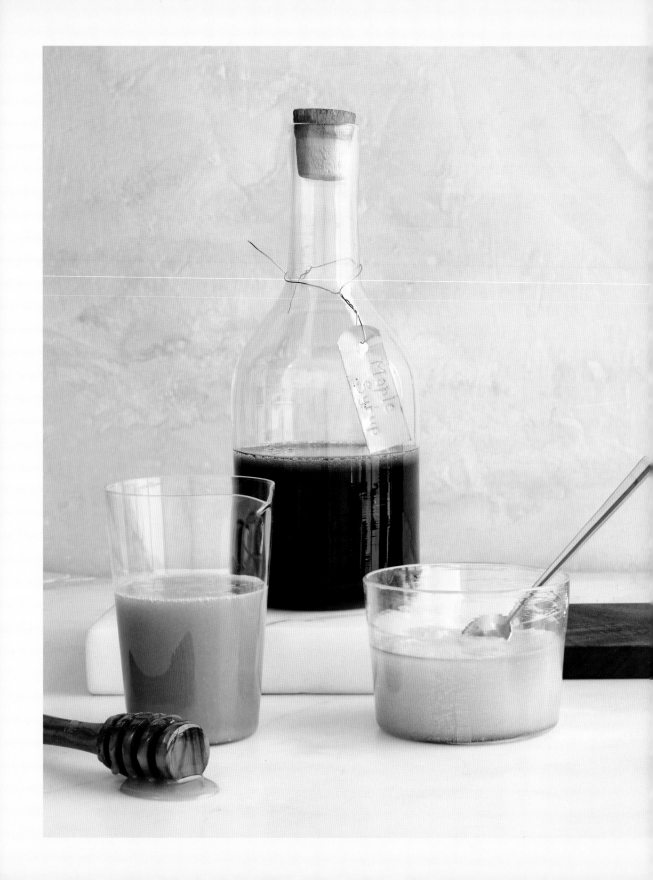

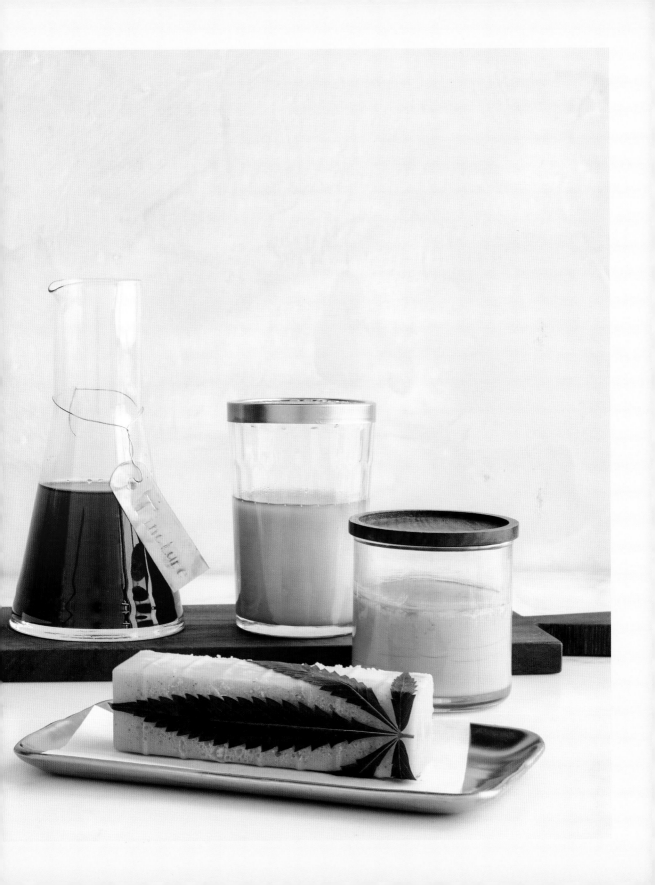

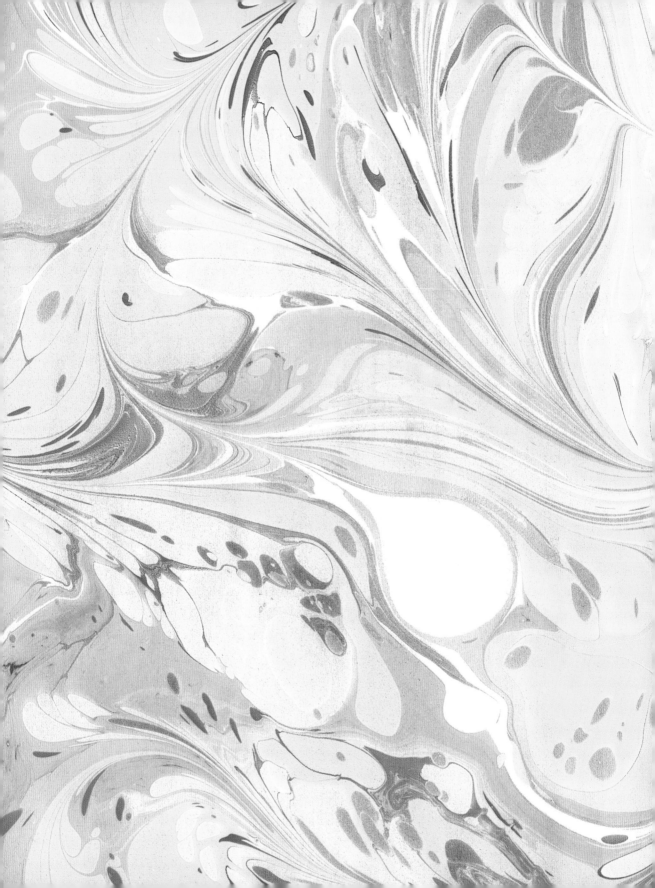

Recipes

EXPLORE, EXPERIMENT,
AND ENJOY!

GF | Gluten Free
DF | Dairy Free

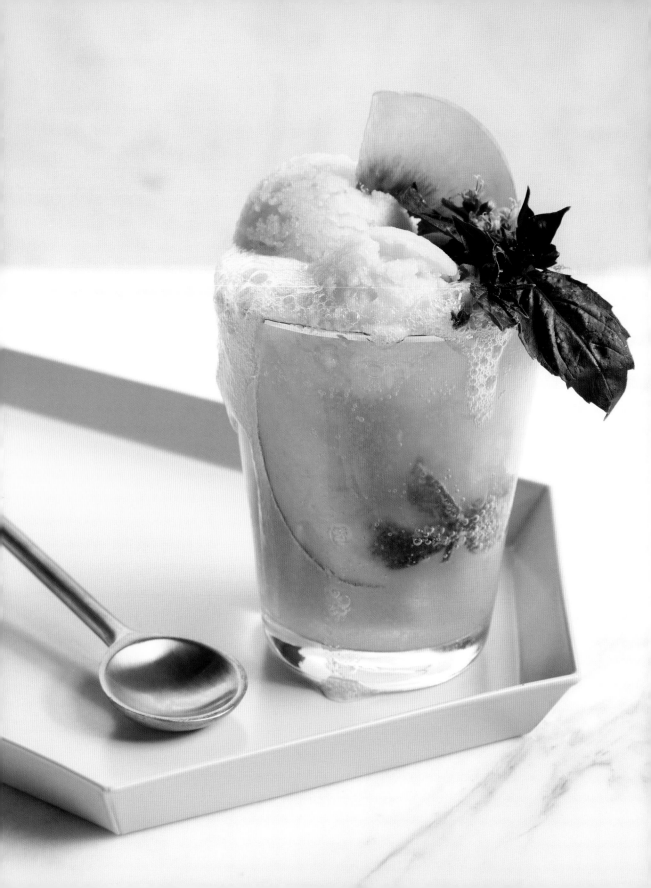

Peach & Ginger Ale Float

| ACTIVE TIME: **10 minutes** | INACTIVE TIME: **0 minutes** | MAKES: **4 floats** |

GF | DF

One 10-oz | 280 g bag frozen peaches or 2 medium peaches, pitted, diced, and frozen

Juice of 2 or 3 limes, depending on how juicy they are

½ tsp | 2 g Canna Tincture (page 33)

1 bunch purple basil or regular basil

32 fl oz | 960 ml ginger ale

Fresh ripe peach slices for garnishing

Take your mocktail game to the next level with this cool and refreshing sorbet float. The sorbet is particularly good in summertime when nectar-sweet, ripe peaches are at the ready. A zing of lime juice perks these up, and fragrant basil adds a subtle floral herbaceousness. If you're lucky enough to find purple basil (sometimes called opal basil), snag it—those deep purple leaves make a spectacular garnish.

In a food processor or blender, combine the frozen peaches and 1 Tbsp lime juice. Blend until the mixture is the consistency of sorbet.

Set out 4 glasses. Place ⅛ tsp [½ g] **canna tincture**, 1 tsp lime juice, and 4 basil leaves into each glass. Using a muddler or the end of a wooden spoon, press down lightly on the leaves until they are fragrant. Fill each glass with ginger ale and stir. Using an ice cream scoop, top each glass with 2 scoops of peach sorbet. Garnish with basil leaves and peach slices. Cheers!

Chocolate Hazelnut Spread

| ACTIVE TIME: **15 minutes** | INACTIVE TIME: **0 minutes** | MAKES: **1½ cups** | **380 g** |

GF

¾ cup | 135 g high-quality semisweet chocolate chips or féves (60% to 65% cacao)

1½ cups | 180 g roasted unsalted hazelnuts, unpeeled is fine

²/₃ cup | 150 g heavy cream

1 Tbsp plus ¾ tsp | 16 g Canna Butter (page 27), at room temperature

Pinch of kosher salt

NOTE

1 serving = 1 Tbsp | 16 g

Be forewarned, you may find yourself sneaking spoonfuls of this sinful chocolate hazelnut spread at all hours of the day (or night!). Slather it on toast or stir a bit into your morning coffee to start the day off right. For heavy hitters who desire stronger dosing, try using this spread in the Banana Cream & Salted Caramel Cookie Cups (page 123), or combine it with Birthday Cake Mellows (page 66) for some killer s'mores.

Place the chocolate in a small heatproof bowl and set aside.

In a food processor, process the hazelnuts for about 5 minutes until you have a loose nut butter, pausing a few times to scrape down the sides of the bowl with a rubber spatula. The nut butter should be fluid enough that it will slowly ooze down like thick molasses if you let it fall from the spatula. Transfer ¼ cup [80 g] to a small saucepan. The remaining nut butter is the chef's snack! (Or freeze the leftover nut butter in an airtight container for up to six months so it's ready to go the next time you want to make this recipe.)

Place the saucepan over medium-high heat and whisk in the cream. Bring the mixture to a simmer, whisking occasionally to combine well and keep the cream from sticking to the bottom of the pan. Once the mixture starts to bubble, immediately remove it from the heat and pour it over the chocolate. Let sit for 3 to 5 minutes until the chocolate melts. Whisk until completely melted and evenly blended.

Add the **canna butter** and salt. Whisk well for about 1 minute to ensure equal distribution of the butter. Scrape down the sides of the bowl with a rubber spatula, and whisk a bit more for good measure. Refrigerate in an airtight container for up to two weeks, or freeze for up to six months.

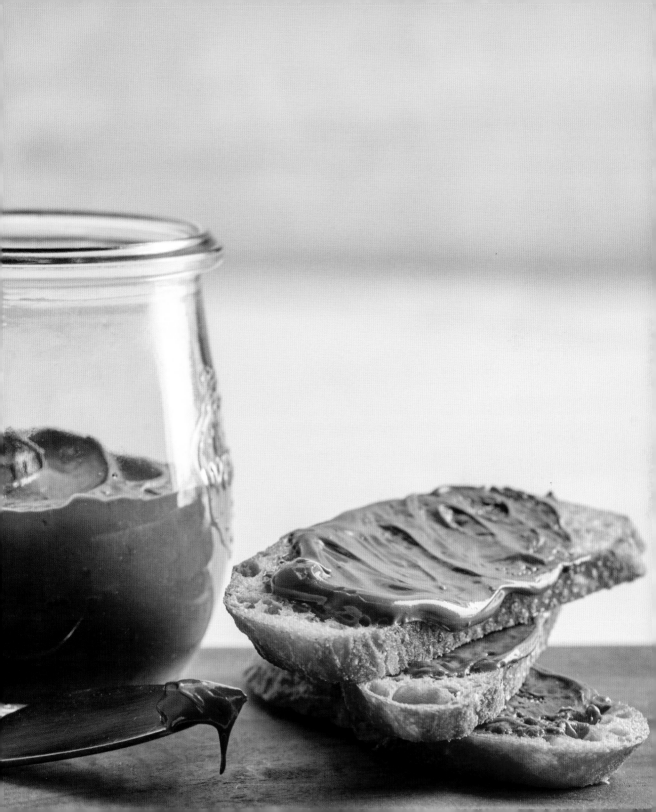

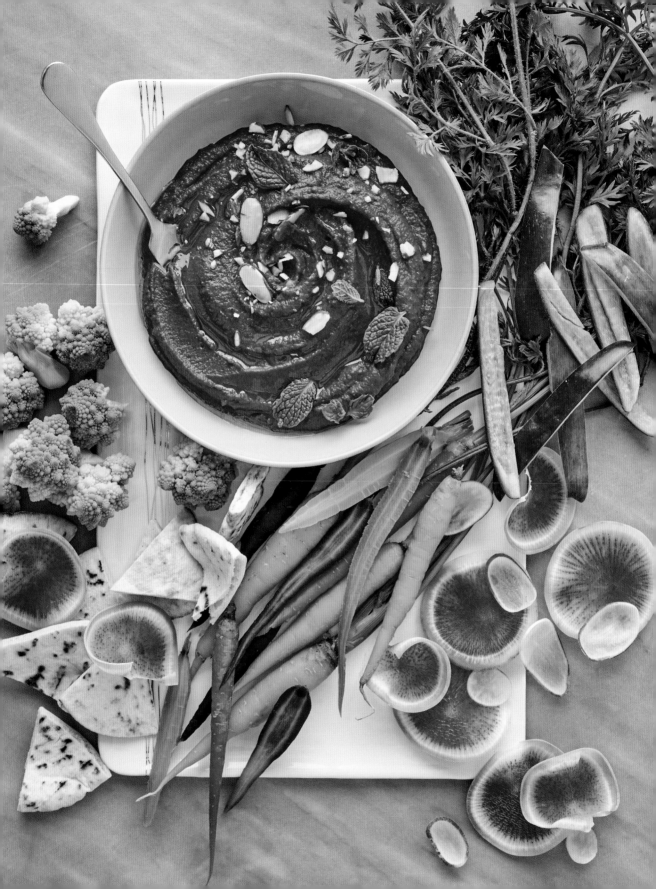

Roasted Beet Hummus

ACTIVE TIME: **15 minutes**	INACTIVE TIME: **30 minutes**	MAKES: **2½ cups** | **680 g**

Roasted beet and garlic bring an unexpected *va va voom* to your ordinary hummus—velvety smooth, earthy, and sweet. Not to mention that color—it's a stunner. Serve with pita chips and crudités, or spread on a sandwich piled high with veggies. If you're into zero waste, save that chickpea liquid (a.k.a. aquafaba) for another use, like making meringues for delightful Strawberry Jam Pavlovas, page 126.

GF | **DF**

10 oz | 280 g beets, about 1 large, washed and ends trimmed

1 head garlic, loose outer layers removed

One 15-oz | 430-g can chickpeas, drained and rinsed

2 Tbsp sliced almonds, plus more for garnishing

⅓ cup | 71 g extra-virgin olive oil, plus more for garnishing

2 Tbsp plus 1½ tsp | 32 g Canna Coconut Oil (page 29)

2½ tsp red wine vinegar, plus more as needed

1½ tsp kosher salt, plus more as needed

¼ tsp freshly ground black pepper, plus more as needed

Fresh mint for garnishing

NOTE

1 serving = 1 Tbsp | 17 g

Preheat the oven to 400°F [200°C].

Wrap the beet in a piece of aluminum foil. Cut about ½ in [12 mm] off the top of the garlic head so the cloves are exposed. Wrap the garlic in foil as well. Place the beet and garlic on a baking sheet and roast for about 30 minutes until the beet is tender enough to pierce easily with a paring knife and the garlic cloves feel soft when pressed. Let the beet cool until you can handle it.

Rub the peel off the cooled beet under running water and cut it into small chunks. Measure out 1¼ cups [200 g] and place it in a food processor (save the remaining beet for another use). Squeeze the roasted garlic cloves out of their skins and into the processor and add the chickpeas, almonds, olive oil, **canna coconut oil**, vinegar, salt, and pepper. Blend for 1 to 2 minutes until smooth and well combined, stopping to scrape down the sides a few times. Taste and season as needed with additional salt, pepper, and vinegar.

Transfer the hummus to a serving bowl. Top with a shower of fresh mint, a sprinkling of sliced almonds, and a healthy lashing of good olive oil.

The hummus can be made ahead and refrigerated in an airtight container for up to three days. Stir well before using.

Carrot Cake Energy Bites

ACTIVE TIME: **20 minutes**	INACTIVE TIME: **45 minutes**	MAKES: **16 2-by-2-in squares**

GF | DF

1 cup | 120 g raw walnut pieces

1 cup | 140 g whole raw almonds

2¾ cups | 220 g unsweetened shredded coconut

1 tsp kosher salt

½ tsp ground cinnamon

½ tsp ground cloves

24 dates | 410 g, pitted

About 2 large | 200 g carrots, cut into ½-in [12-mm] pieces (1⅓ cups)

1 Tbsp | 13 g Canna Coconut Oil (page 29)

2 tsp maple syrup

These healthy, energy-charged bites are perfect when you need a little boost, whether you're running out the door, going for a hike, or craving a midday snack. They're free of dairy, grains, and refined sugar…and yet, they are absolutely scrumptious! Wait, it gets better. Other than toasting nuts, this recipe requires zero cooking. Make these and win at life.

Line an 8-by-8-in [20-by-20-cm] baking pan with plastic wrap and set aside.

In a large skillet over medium-high heat, toast the walnuts and almonds for 3 to 5 minutes until they are lightly browned and fragrant. Transfer to a food processor and add 2½ cups [200g] of the coconut, the salt, cinnamon, and cloves. Process for 20 to 30 seconds into a fine meal.

Add the dates, carrots, **canna coconut oil**, and maple syrup. Process for about 45 seconds until well combined, scraping down the sides of the bowl with a rubber spatula halfway through. The mixture should keep its form when pressed together. Evenly press the mixture into the prepared pan using a pastry scraper or the edge of a spatula. Remember the mixture must be evenly distributed throughout the pan for equal dosing.

Sprinkle the remaining ¼ cup [20 g] of the coconut on top and lightly press into the surface. Freeze until firm, about 45 minutes, but not frozen solid.

Pull up on the edges of the plastic wrap and remove the square from the pan. Cut into 16 equal 2-by-2-in [5-by-5-cm] squares. Keep refrigerated in an airtight container for up to five days, or frozen for up to one month.

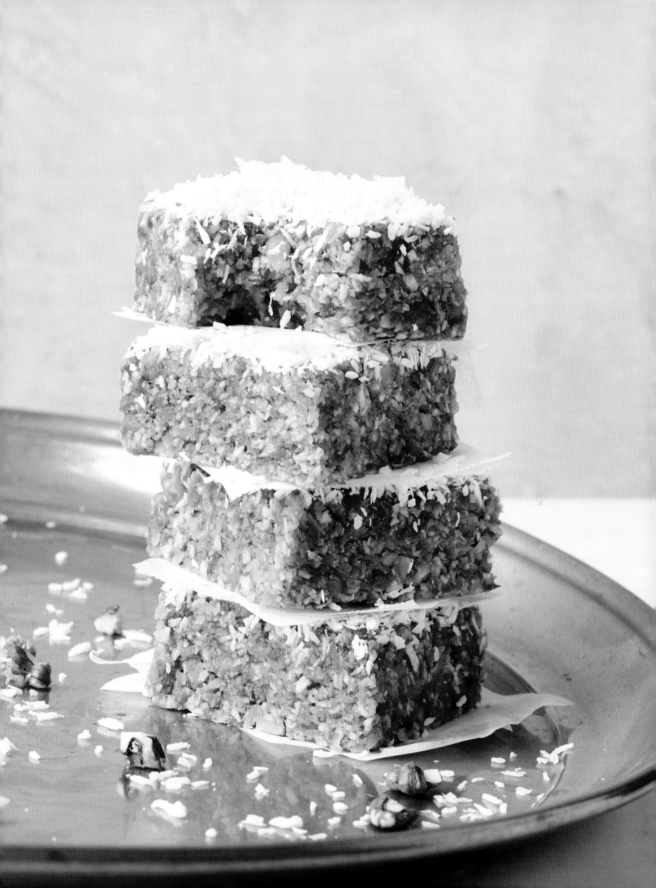

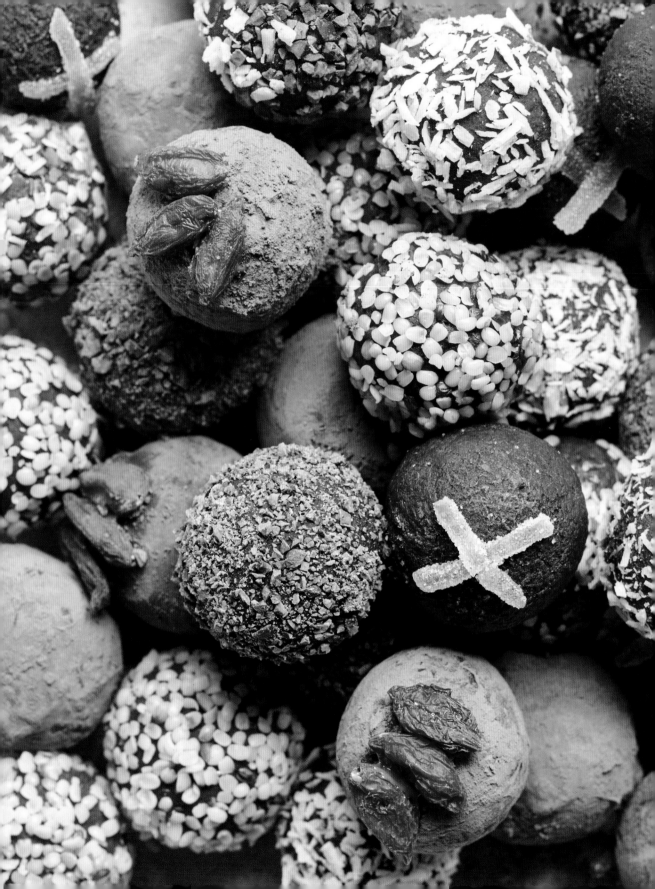

Spiced Superfood Truffles

| ACTIVE TIME: **30 minutes** | INACTIVE TIME: **1 hour** | MAKES: **20 truffles** |

GF | DF

1 ⅓ cups | 240 g high-quality dark chocolate chips or féves (65% to 75% cacao)

¼ cup | 60 g full-fat coconut milk

1 Tbsp plus ¾ tsp | 16 g Canna Coconut Oil (page 29)

½ tsp ground cinnamon

¼ tsp fine sea salt

Pinch of cayenne pepper

SUPERFOOD GARNISHES

Raw hemp hearts (see Note, page 50)

Unsweetened shredded coconut

Raw cacao nibs, finely chopped

Raw cacao powder

Goji berries

Crystallized ginger, finely chopped

SPECIAL EQUIPMENT

Double boiler (page 19)

Cannabis and cacao are two superfoods we would happily consume on the regular. In this recipe, rich coconut milk is used in place of the heavy cream traditionally used to make chocolate truffles, and healthy toppings such as hemp hearts, goji berries, and ginger add a flavor punch along with their nutritional boost. Indulge in these decadent truffles and feel good about doing so! No time to make your own cannabis infusion? Substitute the canna coconut oil in this recipe with one 4-oz [112-g] jar of Whoopi & Maya's Savor Cacao (100 mg THC) and adjust the amount of full-fat coconut milk to 2 Tbsp.

Line an 8-by-8-in [20-by-20-cm] pan with parchment paper (see page 19).

In a medium heatproof bowl set over a double boiler, melt together the chocolate and coconut milk, stirring every so often with a rubber spatula, about 5 minutes.

Add the **canna coconut oil** and stir until well combined and smooth.

Add the cinnamon, salt, and cayenne. Stir to combine. Pour the chocolate mixture into the prepared pan, using the spatula to scrape out every last bit. Use an offset spatula or pastry scraper to spread the chocolate into an even layer.

Refrigerate the chocolate for about 1 hour until firm enough to cut and form. While you wait, prepare your superfood garnishes of choice and separate them in small bowls. Line a baking sheet with parchment and set aside.

CONT'D

Hemp hearts are not only nutritious, but they are also delicious with a subtle, nutty flavor.

Remove the chocolate from the pan by lifting the parchment. Cut the chocolate into twenty equal (2-by-1⅝ -in [5-by-4-cm]) pieces. Using your palms, roll each piece into a ball and place it on the prepared sheet. If the chocolate starts to get melty and hard to work with, pop it back into the fridge to firm up.

Roll the truffle balls in the garnishes and return to the sheet. If using the larger garnishes, such as the goji berries and ginger, roll the truffle first in cacao powder and press just a few pieces of the garnish on top. Refrigerate the coated truffles for about 15 minutes to set.

Pack the truffles in an airtight container with wax paper or parchment between each layer, and refrigerate for up to two weeks, or freeze for up to three months. Let the truffles warm for 5 to 10 minutes at room temperature before enjoying.

MAKER PROFILE

Whoopi Goldberg and Maya Elisabeth
Whoopi & Maya

Whoopi Goldberg and Maya Elisabeth are the powerhouse team behind Whoopi & Maya, a line of cannabis products designed specifically to provide relief for women during their moon cycles—from cramping and pain to irritability. Whoopi and Maya treat cannabis as what it truly is for many people—powerful herbal medicine.

"I believe cannabis is a superfood," says Maya. "And when cannabis is combined with other healing herbs and nutrient-dense ingredients, a superior medicine is made." It is no wonder that Savor, Whoopi & Maya's raw cacao product, is so effective. Raw chocolate is rich in antioxidants, magnesium, and iron. It stimulates the release of serotonin and endorphins, both associated with feelings of comfort and happiness. "When I found that out I laughed so hard," Maya said. "I mean, how many times have I gone to chocolate for comfort? What woman hasn't? The word *cacao* even means gift from the gods!"

On top of all that, fascinatingly enough, cacao is one of the few foods that contain cannabinoids, chemical compounds that enter your body through your endocannabinoid receptors—just like cannabis—and release an array of feel-good chemicals that physically improve your mood.

So, you see, cannabis and chocolate were meant to be together. And, those chocolate cravings you get? They are legit and you should satisfy them.

Green Eggs & Ham

| ACTIVE TIME: **35 minutes** | INACTIVE TIME: **15 minutes** | MAKES: **12 egg & ham cups** |

CONT'D

EGG & HAM CUPS

8 oz | 230 g thinly sliced prosciutto

12 large eggs, at room temperature

Freshly ground black pepper

1 garlic clove, minced

12 tsp | 29 g grated Parmigiano-Reggiano cheese

Wake n' bake done right. We would eat these here or there; we would eat these anywhere. These adorable, conveniently portioned egg cups are the perfect brunch offering. If you have access to fresh cannabis leaves, they make a great addition to the herb pesto here—which, by the way, can be used a hundred different ways on its own. Spread it on a sandwich, dollop it over grilled meat, or stir some into pasta or cheesy grits. Oh, the possibilities...

Preheat the oven to 375°F [190°C].

TO MAKE THE EGG & HAM CUPS: Line each muffin pan cup with 1 to 1½ slices of prosciutto, making sure to cover the entire bottom and sides of the cup. The prosciutto will shrink a bit as it cooks, so be generous with the amount of area it covers and don't try to stretch it.

Crack 1 egg into each cup. Top each egg with a crack of freshly ground pepper, a pinch of minced garlic, and 1 tsp of grated Parmigiano cheese. Bake for 10 to 12 minutes until the whites have set but the yolks are still runny. If you like your yolks firmer, bake for up to 5 minutes more. While the eggs cook, prepare the herb pesto.

CONT'D

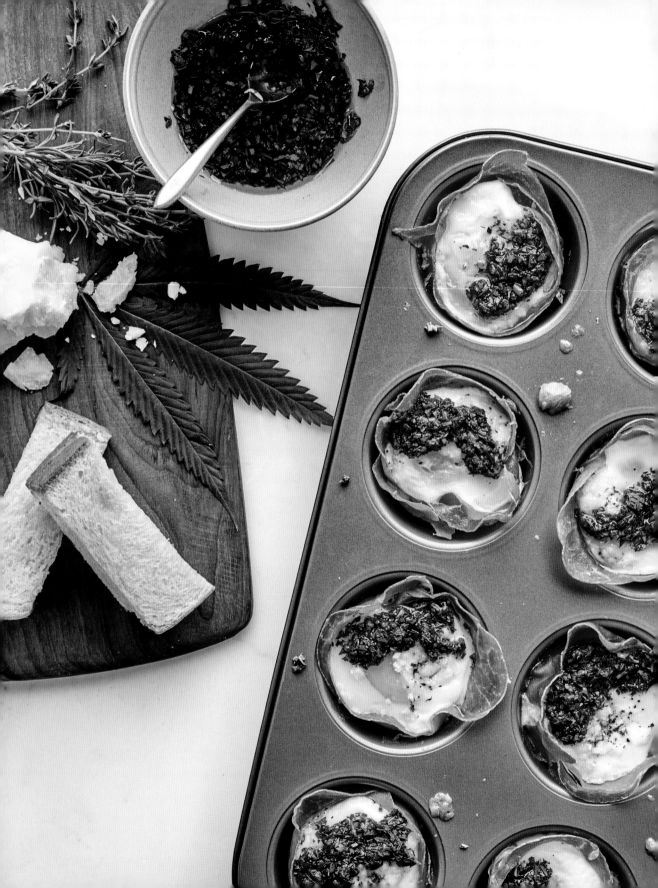

½ cup | 40 g packed fresh cannabis leaves or parsley leaves, finely chopped

1 Tbsp fresh thyme leaves, finely chopped

1 Tbsp fresh rosemary leaves, finely chopped

Zest of ½ lemon

½ tsp kosher salt

¼ tsp freshly ground black pepper

2¼ tsp | 10 g Canna Coconut Oil (page 29), melted

½ cup | 108 g extra-virgin olive oil

ON THE SIDE

Toast points or buttered and griddled brioche sticks for serving

SPECIAL EQUIPMENT

12-cup muffin pan

TO MAKE THE HERB PESTO: In a liquid measuring cup, combine the cannabis leaves, thyme, rosemary, lemon zest, salt, and pepper. Stir in the **canna coconut oil** until well combined. Scrape down the sides of the cup with a rubber spatula. Add enough olive oil to the measuring cup to reach the ¾-cup [180-ml] mark. With a fork or small whisk, stir the pesto vigorously to combine thoroughly. Evenly divide the pesto among the egg cups—1 level Tbsp pesto per cup. Stir the pesto as needed so each spoonful has an equal amount of herbs and oil.

Serve with toast points or buttered and griddled brioche sticks to sop up all the goodness.

Roasted Grape Crostini

ACTIVE TIME: **20 minutes** | INACTIVE TIME: **35 minutes** | MAKES: **18 crostini**

These crostini are the perfect party bite. They hit just the right balance between savory and sweet, creamy and crunchy—and those roasted grapes: game changing. It may seem unorthodox to roast grapes, but trust us on this. The roasting concentrates and develops the sugar in the fruit, resulting in a caramelized, complex sweetness. It's the perfect counter to the savory mascarpone-cashew cream spread, which is also slightly unusual, but completely delicious.

ROASTED GRAPES

1 lb | 455 g seedless red grapes

1 Tbsp extra-virgin olive oil

½ tsp kosher salt

¼ tsp freshly ground black pepper

4 sprigs thyme, halved widthwise

2 sprigs rosemary, halved widthwise

CASHEW CREAM

⅔ cup | 153 g mascarpone cheese

2 Tbsp cashew butter

2¾ tsp | 12 g Canna Butter (page 27), at room temperature

½ tsp kosher salt

CONT'D

Preheat the oven to 400°F [200°C]. Line a sheet pan with parchment paper.

TO MAKE THE ROASTED GRAPES: On the prepared sheet pan, toss together the grapes, olive oil, salt, pepper, thyme, and rosemary. Roast for about 30 minutes until the grapes are blistered and jammy, stirring once halfway through. Remove and set aside.

TO MAKE THE CASHEW CREAM: In the bowl of a stand mixer fitted with the paddle attachment, or in a large bowl with a handheld mixer, combine the mascarpone, cashew butter, **canna butter**, and salt. Whip for about 30 seconds on medium speed until well combined. Do not overbeat or your mixture can separate.

CONT'D

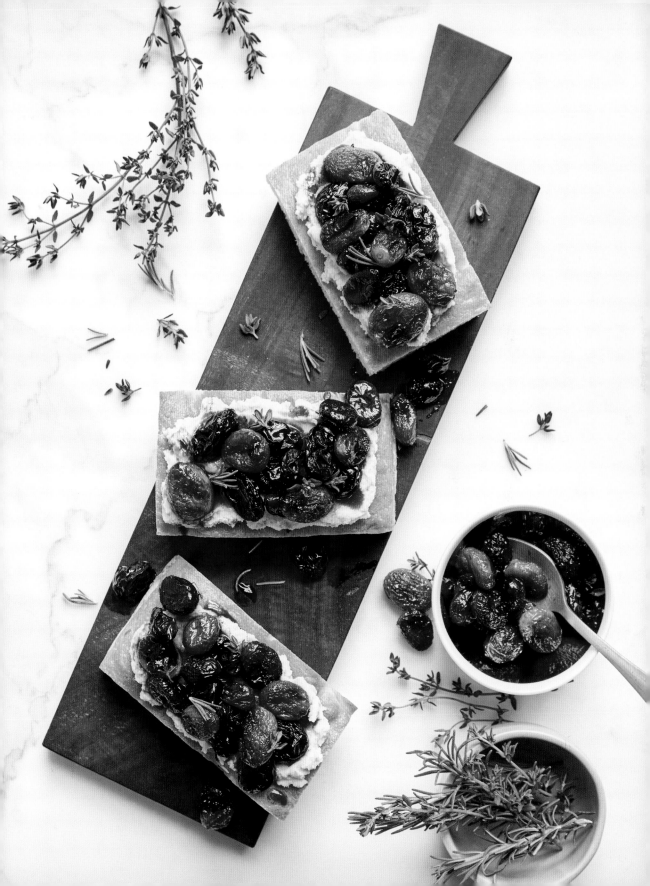

One 8-by-12-in
[20-by-30.5-cm]
loaf focaccia bread

Extra-virgin olive oil
for brushing the crostini

Kosher salt

Freshly ground black pepper

MAKE-AHEAD TIP

The roasted grapes can be made
ahead and kept refrigerated in an
airtight container for up to three
days. Warm before using.

TO MAKE THE CROSTINI: Preheat the broiler to high.

Split the focaccia in half like a big sandwich bun. Cut the top and
bottom halves into 3 rows, then cut each row into 3 pieces. You
should have a total of 18 pieces measuring about 2½ in by 4 in [6 cm
by 10 cm]. With a pastry brush, brush the cut side of the focaccia
pieces with olive oil and season with salt and pepper. Place the
crostini on a baking sheet and under the broiler for 3 to 5 minutes
until lightly golden.

TO ASSEMBLE: Spread 2 tsp cashew cream onto each crostini
and top with a spoonful of roasted grapes. Drizzle any *jus* from the
grapes and enjoy immediately.

The Elvis Cookie

ACTIVE TIME: **40 minutes**	INACTIVE TIME: **30 minutes**	MAKES: **16 cookies**

6 Tbsp | 85 g unsalted butter

½ cup | 90 g high-quality semisweet chocolate chips (60% to 65% cacao)

2 ¾ tsp | 12 g Canna Butter (page 27), at room temperature

½ cup | 100 g packed light brown sugar

½ cup | 70 g all-purpose flour

¼ cup plus 2 Tbsp | 30 g unsweetened cocoa powder

¼ tsp baking soda

¼ tsp kosher salt

1 large egg, at room temperature

1 tsp vanilla extract

½ cup | 42 g banana chips, roughly chopped

½ cup | 85 g peanut butter chips

¼ cup | 45 g white chocolate chips

SPECIAL EQUIPMENT
Double boiler (page 19)

The Venice Cookie Company calls their Elvis Cookie the King of Cookies, clocking in at a mighty 1,000 mg THC per cookie. We've adapted their original recipe here, bringing the dosage way down for us plebs, but keeping all the other good stuff intact, like chocolate chips, peanut butter chips, and banana chips. We'd like to think this treat would inspire a few shake, rattle, and rolls from the King of Rock 'n' Roll himself.

Preheat the oven to 325°F [165°C]. Line 2 baking sheets with parchment paper or silicone baking mats.

In a medium heatproof bowl over a double boiler, melt together the butter and semisweet chocolate, stirring every so often with a rubber spatula, about 5 minutes.

Add the **canna butter** and whisk to combine. Whisk in the brown sugar, remove from the heat, and let cool for about 5 minutes.

Meanwhile, in a medium bowl, whisk the flour, cocoa powder, baking soda, and salt. Set aside.

Whisk the egg and vanilla into the chocolate mixture.

Add half the flour mixture to the chocolate mixture and fold to combine. Fold in the remaining flour mixture.

Add the banana chips, peanut butter chips, and white chocolate chips, and fold again until just combined. Do not overmix.

CONT'D

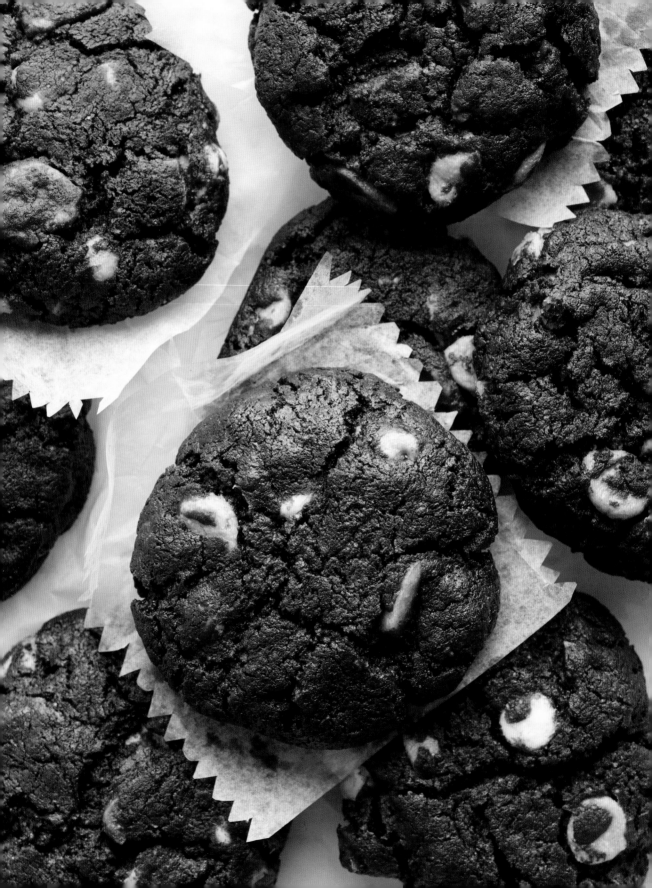

The cookie dough can be made, portioned, flattened, and frozen, then stored in an airtight container in the freezer for up to three months. Bake as directed directly from the freezer.

VARIATION

To make a double-dose Elvis Cookie sandwich, sandwich peanut butter and fresh banana slices between two cookies! Crumble in some candied bacon to pay true homage to the King. (Elvis was known to throw some bacon into his fried peanut butter and banana sandwiches when he was feeling especially kinglike.)

Refrigerate the dough for about 15 minutes to rest and firm up.

Weigh the dough and divide into sixteen equal balls. Using a scale to portion the dough is highly recommended for this recipe, however, if you do not have a scale, portion the dough using a 2-Tbsp [30-ml] cookie scoop, or 2 level Tbsp [30 ml] per cookie. If you go this route, level the scoop when measuring and scrape out all the dough completely from the scoop each time.

Place eight dough balls onto each of the prepared sheets, spacing them evenly so they have room to spread. Press them down slightly to flatten. Bake for 12 to 15 minutes until the cookies are dry on the surface, but still a little soft on the inside. Let the cookies cool on the baking sheet. They will firm up once completely cooled, but we can't resist indulging in these while they are still warm and gooey!

MAKER PROFILE

Kenny Morrison
Venice Cookie Company

In 2008 Kenny Morrison started Venice Cookie Company with three homemade cookie recipes. He called it Venice Cookie Company because of what the people and community of Venice, California, have always stood for—individuality, creativity, rebellious and radical innovation, and self-expression.

"The Venice boardwalk is probably the closest thing Southern California has ever had to a Haight-Ashbury," Kenny says. "I've always been honored to pay respect to the Bay Area as the birthplace of medical cannabis, how it jump-started the movement toward normalization and legalization, with significant contributions made by the gay community in the early years. I think the same ethos and fiery passion found on the streets of San Francisco in those days can be found on the streets of Venice as well."

Kenny admits, "Venice had more mystique and allure back in the day before all the money moved in, and I miss it. All things evolve, nothing stays the same, but Venice Cookie Company will always stand for the deeply held beliefs that have defined it from the beginning—that the status quo should always be challenged in the pursuit of finding a better way. Peace. Love. Cannabis."

And cookies . . . always cookies.

Apple Power Crumble

| ACTIVE TIME: **30 minutes** | INACTIVE TIME: **40 minutes** | MAKES: **6 servings** |

The ladies at Treat Yourself are experts at creating healthy and wholesome edibles that taste great and are great for you. This apple crumble is no exception. Sweetened with nothing but a touch of Canna Honey (page 34), and topped with a nutritious, toasty crumble of oats, coconut, seeds, and hemp hearts, this healthy treat will power you through the day. Apples not in season? Berries and stone fruit make a fine substitution. Don't want to fuss with a filling at all? Bake the crumble on a sheet pan and call it granola.

GF | DF

APPLE FILLING

2 lb | 910 g apples, 5 to 6 medium, unpeeled, cored, and diced into ½-in [12-mm] pieces

2 Tbsp water

1 tsp vanilla extract

½ tsp ground cinnamon

Zest of 1 orange

POWER CRUMBLE TOPPING

2 Tbsp plus ¾ tsp | 41 g Canna Honey (page 34)

¼ cup | 55 g coconut oil, melted

1 cup | 100 g old-fashioned rolled oats (gluten free)

½ cup | 40 g shredded unsweetened coconut

1 Tbsp chia seeds

1 Tbsp white sesame seeds

1 Tbsp raw pepitas (shelled pumpkin seeds)

CONT'D

Preheat the oven to 325°F [165°C].

TO MAKE THE APPLE FILLING: In a large saucepan over medium heat, combine the apples, water, vanilla, cinnamon, and orange zest. Cook for 15 to 20 minutes, stirring occasionally, until the apples have completely softened.

TO MAKE THE POWER CRUMBLE TOPPING: In a small microwave-safe container, slightly warm the **canna honey** for 10 to 20 seconds so it is pourable. Transfer to a medium bowl and add the coconut oil. Whisk until well combined. Add the remaining crumble topping ingredients and mix well.

CONT'D

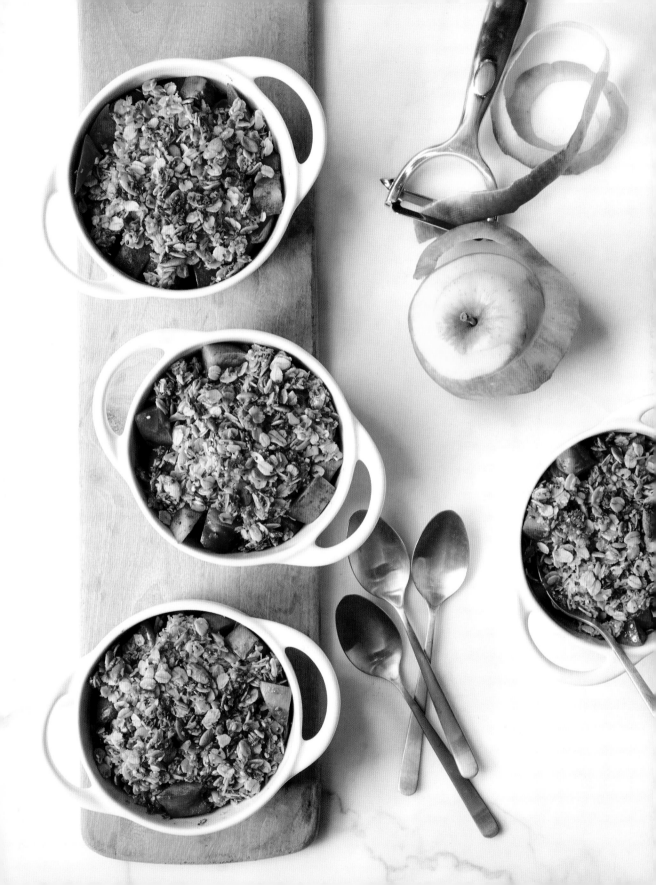

1 Tbsp hemp hearts

1 tsp vanilla extract

½ tsp kosher salt

½ tsp ground cinnamon

MAKE-AHEAD TIP

The crumble can be made ahead, stored in an airtight container, and frozen for up to one month.

TO ASSEMBLE: Place six 8-fl oz [240-ml] baking dishes or wide-mouth glass Mason jars on a sturdy rimmed baking sheet. Divide the apple mixture equally (about ⅔ cup [80 g] apple mixture per serving) among the baking dishes.

Top each with an equal amount of the crumble mixture, about ⅓ cup [50 g]. For the most accurate dosage, weigh the total amount of medicated crumble and divide by six to determine the target weight per serving.

Bake for 35 to 40 minutes until the crumble is golden and toasty, rotating the tray halfway through the baking time. Serve warm.

MAKER PROFILE

Leone Posod and Cindy Pinzon
Treat Yourself

Longtime childhood friends Leone Posod and Cindy Pinzon are the ladies behind Treat Yourself, a company that specializes in creating healthy cannabis-infused products with women in mind.

For Leone and Cindy, treating yourself and treating yourself right are not mutually exclusive. "We want to show people that something can be delicious and enjoyable, and good for you at the same time," says Cindy.

That means nutrient-rich edibles made from high-quality, organic ingredients sourced from nature: edibles such as their mini pop tartelettes, made with chia seed dough and real fruit; or paleo banana bread; or apple crumble topped with a mix of power foods such as hemp hearts, seeds, and coconut. All the treats Leone and Cindy make are vegan, gluten free, and refined sugar free.

"Our mission with Treat Yourself is to cultivate health and happiness," says Leone. "We are big proponents of self-care, and believe that cannabis not only treats a plethora of ailments, it also helps us tune in to more subtle messages from our bodies."

Cindy adds, "We also believe in the power of food as medicine. In our everyday diet we try to incorporate as many nutrient-packed foods as possible. It only made sense to translate that to our edibles." Which is why you won't see anything in the ingredient list you can't pronounce.

This wholesome Apple Power Crumble is proof that you can treat yourself while treating yourself right. If this is what healthy tastes like, sign us up!

Pimiento Cheese &
Tomato Tea Sandwiches

| ACTIVE TIME: **30 minutes** | INACTIVE TIME: **0 minutes** | MAKES: **24 servings** |

4 oz | 115 g cream cheese, at room temperature

One 2-oz | 55-g can diced pimientos, drained

3 Tbsp | 45 g mayonnaise

2 Tbsp miso paste

1 Tbsp plus 1½ tsp | 19 g Canna Coconut Oil (page 29), at room temperature

¼ tsp garlic powder

¼ tsp onion powder

Pinch of cayenne pepper

Pinch of freshly ground black pepper

½ cup | 25 g loosely packed grated Gruyère cheese

1 cup | 45 g loosely packed grated sharp Cheddar cheese

Kosher salt

3 medium heirloom tomatoes (preferably in 3 different colors)

6 slices sandwich bread

Fresh basil leaves for garnishing

This modern twist on the traditional pimiento sandwich is one of our favorite items to serve at "high" tea events and potluck picnics, especially in summertime when tomatoes are at their sweetest. It is hard to decide who's the star of the show here—the umami-rich, miso-laced cheese spread or that gorgeous tomato mosaic. Don't let the long ingredient list deter you—this comes together quickly and the fun you'll have serving this throwback number is worth it.

In the bowl of a stand mixer fitted with the paddle attachment, or in a large bowl with a handheld mixer, combine the cream cheese, pimientos, mayonnaise, miso, **canna coconut oil**, garlic powder, onion powder, cayenne, and black pepper. Beat for about 1 minute on medium speed until all the ingredients are thoroughly combined. Scrape down the sides and bottom of the bowl and beat once more.

Using a rubber spatula, fold in the Gruyère and Cheddar cheeses, mixing until well combined. Make sure you incorporate all the way from the bottom and up the sides of the bowl. Season with salt, as desired.

Using a serrated knife, cut the tomatoes into thin slices (⅛ to ¼ in [4 to 6 mm] thick). If the tomatoes are very large, halve them vertically before slicing. Place the tomato slices on paper towels to absorb some of the juices.

CONT'D

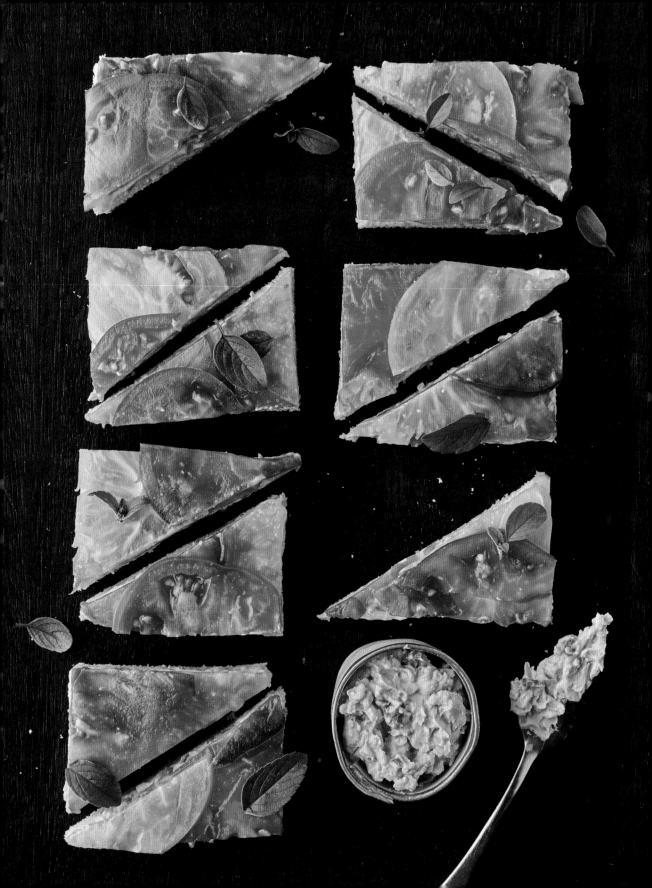

Lay out the bread slices. Spread each piece with an equal amount of cheese spread, about 3 packed Tbsp [49 g], avoiding the edges where the crusts will be cut off. For the most accurate dosage, weigh the total amount of cheese spread and divide by six to determine the amount of spread per slice.

Arrange 3 or 4 tomato slices on top, partially overlapping and alternating colors. Cut off the crusts. With the long side facing you, halve each piece of bread vertically, then on the diagonal, so you end up with four equal triangles.

Garnish with fresh basil, admire your tomato mosaic, and enjoy immediately.

Birthday Cake Mellows

ACTIVE TIME: **30 minutes**　　INACTIVE TIME: **24 hours**　　MAKES: **36 bite-size squares**

So fluffy and light, you may just float away! Once you've tried homemade marshmallows, you'll never look at that store-bought package the same way again. The hardest part of making these is waiting for them to set. These Mellows pack big fun in a little bite. Enjoy them in homemade s'mores, ice cream sundaes, hot chocolate, or coffee!

GF | DF

2 packets | 14 g unflavored powdered gelatin

¾ cup | 180 g water

1½ cups | 300 g sugar

¾ cup plus 1 Tbsp | 260 g light corn syrup

½ tsp kosher salt

2 Tbsp plus ¾ tsp | 29 g Canna Coconut Oil (page 29), melted

2 tsp vanilla extract

½ cup | 80 g rainbow sprinkles

½ cup | 70 g cornstarch

½ cup | 60 g powdered sugar

SPECIAL EQUIPMENT

Instant-read thermometer or candy thermometer

Spray an 8-by-8-in [20-by-20-cm] baking pan with nonstick baking spray.

In the bowl of a stand mixer fitted with the whisk attachment, combine the gelatin and ½ cup [120 g] of the water. Stir until the gelatin is hydrated and there are no large clumps. Set aside.

In a medium saucepan over high heat, combine the sugar, corn syrup, remaining ¼ cup [60 g] of water, and salt. (If using a candy thermometer, clip it to the saucepan.) Without stirring, bring the mixture to 240°F [115°C], about 5 minutes. (If using an instant-read thermometer, check the temperature by tilting the pan so the probe measures the temperature of the syrup and not the bottom of the pan. The syrup will be bubbling aggressively so be careful.) Remove the mixture from the heat and cool to 220°F [105°C], stirring with a rubber spatula in a figure-eight motion to speed the cooling, about 5 minutes.

CONT'D

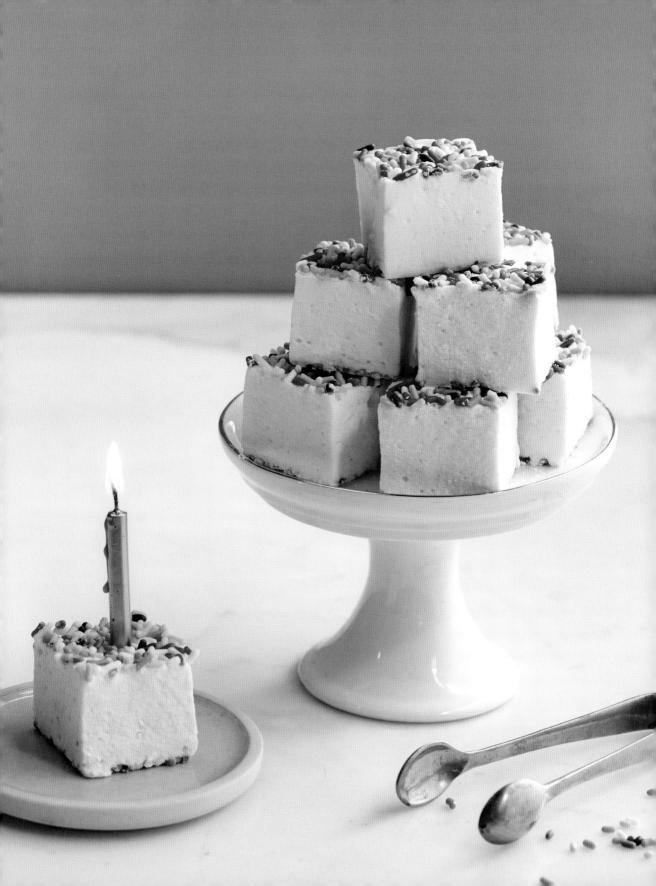

Carefully pour the sugar syrup into the bloomed gelatin in the mixer bowl. Using the whisk attachment, beat the mixture for about 10 minutes on medium-high speed until thick and gooey. Turn the speed to low, and, with the mixer running, drizzle in the **canna coconut oil**. Add the vanilla, crank the speed to high, and whisk for about 2 minutes until the mixture is voluminous and light as a cloud. Scrape down the sides of the bowl with a rubber spatula, as needed.

Cover the bottom of the prepared baking pan with half the rainbow sprinkles. Pour the fluffy marshmallow mixture into the pan. Use a rubber spatula to scrape as much as possible from the bowl. It will be sticky and messy, but do your best (if you are tempted to lick your fingers, just remember this is "special" batter!). Use an offset spatula or pastry scraper to spread the marshmallow evenly in the pan, or tilt the pan to get it into the corners. Smack the pan down on the counter a few times to break any air bubbles. Pop any stubborn bubbles with a toothpick or the tip of a paring knife. Cover the top with the remaining sprinkles—let it rain!

Let sit, uncovered, at room temperature, for 24 hours.

In a large bowl, sift together the cornstarch and powdered sugar. Turn the marshmallow out of the pan by flipping the pan upside-down and using your fingers to pry the edges loose. Use the edge of your hand to work the rest of it out. The marshmallow slab should be upside down on your work surface now. Dust it with the cornstarch-powdered sugar mixture and flip it right-side up. Coat a sharp knife with baking spray. Cut the slab into 36 equal squares. Roll the cut edges in the cornstarch-powdered sugar mix to keep them from sticking to one another when you store them.

Store in an airtight container at room temperature for up to one month, or freeze for up to six months.

Coconut Yogurt & Honeycomb

ACTIVE TIME: **30 minutes**	INACTIVE TIME: **12 to 24 hours**	MAKES: **8 3-oz** | **85-g servings**

This homemade coconut yogurt is so creamy and luxurious it could be dessert. Using organic, higher quality, coconut milk results in the best-tasting yogurt. We dressed it up with crispy honeycomb candy and fragrant fennel notes for a more elegant plating, but it would be just as delightful served as breakfast with your favorite granola and fresh berries. Or, use the yogurt to make medicated smoothies or mango lassi!

GF | **DF**

COCONUT YOGURT

Two 13½-fl oz | 400 ml cans full-fat organic coconut milk

2 Tbsp tapioca starch

One 5-g packet nondairy yogurt starter (see Note, page 71)

2 Tbsp plus 2 tsp | 50 g Canna Maple Syrup (page 35)

HONEYCOMB

½ cup | 170 g honey

¼ cup | 60 g warm water

1¼ cups | 250 g sugar

1 Tbsp baking soda

FINISHING TOUCHES

Fennel pollen for garnishing (see Note, page 71)

Fennel fronds or flowers for garnishing (optional)

SPECIAL EQUIPMENT

1-qt [960-ml] glass Mason jar with lid

Instant-read thermometer or candy thermometer

TO MAKE THE COCONUT YOGURT: Fill the 1-qt jar [960-ml] with boiling water to sterilize it. Place the lid in a bowl and pour boiling water over it to sterilize as well. Let the water stand for at least 5 minutes before pouring it out.

Shake the cans of coconut milk well so the cream on top is mixed in with the milk. In a small bowl, whisk ⅓ cup [80 ml] coconut milk and the tapioca starch until well combined. This step is important to ensure the starch mixes evenly with the milk without clumping.

Into a very clean medium saucepan over medium heat, pour the remaining coconut milk from the open can and add the second can. (If using a candy thermometer, clip it to the saucepan.) Add the starch mixture to the saucepan, making sure to scrape out the bowl, and bring it to 180°F [82°C] over medium heat, whisking occasionally, 5 to 7 minutes. (If using an instant-read thermometer, check the temperature by tilting the pan so the probe measures the temperature of the liquid and not the bottom of the pan.) Remove from the heat and let cool to 110°F [43°C], whisking occasionally to help cool the mixture, about 30 minutes.

CONT'D

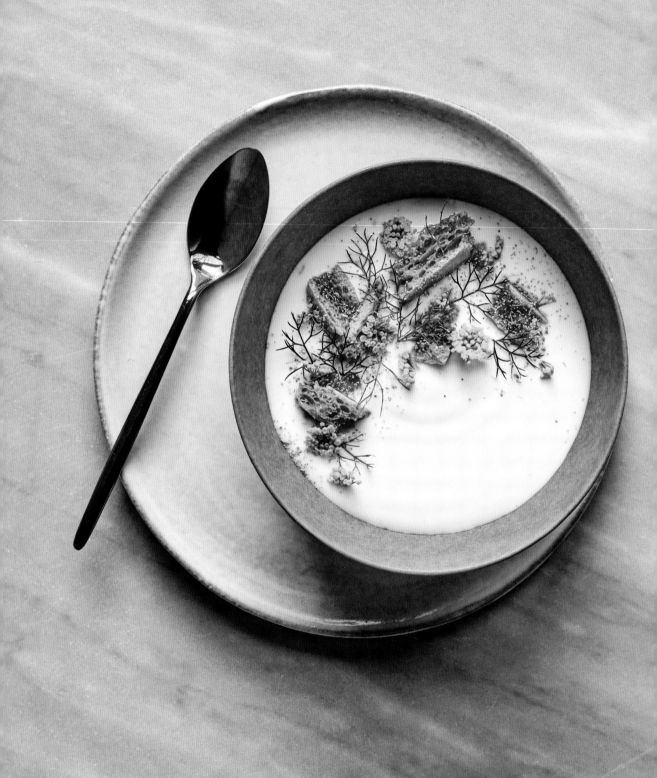

It is important that all the utensils and equipment used in this recipe are very clean and free of any food residue because of the sensitive nature of this fermentation process, and so the yogurt starter develops properly.

Since coconut milk is the base of this yogurt, make sure your yogurt starter culture is *nondairy*. We use Belle+Bella nondairy yogurt starter.

Fennel pollen is a prized spice harvested from tiny fennel flowers. Fragrant with sweet licorice notes, a little bit goes a long way.

Meanwhile, preheat the oven to 100°F [35°C]. When it reaches temperature, turn off the heat and leave the light on to help keep the oven warm.

In a liquid measuring cup, measure ⅓ cup [80 ml] of the coconut milk mixture. Add the yogurt starter and whisk to combine. Pour this mixture back into the saucepan and stir in the **canna maple syrup**. Mix well.

Pour the yogurt mixture into the sterilized jar and seal with the lid. Place the jar in the warmed oven with the light on. Alternatively, use a yogurt maker or place in a dehydrator at 110°F [43°C]. Leave the yogurt undisturbed for 12 to 24 hours. Check it after 12 hours. Using a clean, stainless steel spoon, stir and taste the yogurt for tartness. The longer the yogurt cultures, the tangier it becomes. Taste it every few hours after the 12-hour mark. When the flavor is to your liking (our sweet spot is typically around 14 hours), refrigerate the yogurt for at least 6 hours to thicken.

TO MAKE THE HONEYCOMB: Line a baking sheet with parchment paper or a silicone baking mat and lightly coat it with nonstick baking spray. Place it next to the stovetop. Have a whisk and rubber spatula ready.

In a liquid measuring cup, stir together the honey and warm water (warm from the tap is fine, you just don't want it to be cold or the honey will seize up and be hard to stir). Place the sugar in a large (at least 4-qt [3.8-L]) saucepan. Pour the honey and water mixture into the center of the pan. The sugar will absorb the liquid. Place the saucepan over medium-high heat. Bring the mixture to 300°F [150°C] without stirring, about 10 minutes. If some syrup splashes up the sides of the pan, wash it down using a pastry brush dipped in water.

Remove the pan from the heat. Briskly whisk in the baking soda until it's incorporated (the mixture will bubble up and foam wildly) and immediately pour the mixture onto the prepared baking sheet, without spreading. Use a rubber spatula to scrape out all the honeycomb mixture. Set aside to cool for 20 to 30 minutes. Cut into roughly 2-in [5-cm] pieces. Transfer to an airtight container (this candy is prone to absorbing moisture from the air and turning into a sticky mess). Reserve for garnishing.

CONT'D

For a stronger dose, add a drizzle of Canna Honey (page 34) on top.

TO ASSEMBLE: Give the yogurt a good stir and divide equally among eight bowls or small jars (4-fl oz [120 ml] glass jelly jars work well since each portion will be about 3 oz [85 g]). For the most accurate dosage, weigh the total amount of yogurt and divide by eight to determine the target weight per serving. Cut the honeycomb candy into small, irregularly shaped shards. Garnish the yogurt cups with a few pieces of candy, a pinch of fennel pollen, and a wisp of fennel frond.

Refrigerate any leftover coconut yogurt in a sealed jar for up to two weeks. Store honeycomb candy in an airtight container at room temperature for up to three days. If you have any food-grade desiccant packets, throw a few in to help extend the candy's storage.

Cardamom Caramels

| ACTIVE TIME: **35 minutes** | INACTIVE TIME: **3 hours** | MAKES: **48 2-by-1-in pieces** |

GF

1 cup | 240 g heavy cream

1½ Tbsp | 22 g unsalted butter

2 Tbsp plus 1½ tsp | 32 g Canna Butter (page 27)

1 tsp ground cardamom

1 Tbsp kosher salt

¼ cup | 80 g light corn syrup

¼ cup | 60 g water

1½ cups | 300 g sugar

1 tsp vanilla bean paste or vanilla extract

SPECIAL EQUIPMENT
Instant-read thermometer or candy thermometer

These chewy caramels have just the right amount of salt and a touch of cardamom to give them an aromatic allure. Pack them in a pretty tin to make an unforgettable gift. This recipe makes a generous number of caramels, so don't feel guilty keeping a few for yourself. Once you've mastered this technique, you may find yourself making batch after batch. Get creative with the flavor profile and try swapping pumpkin spice, ground ginger, or espresso powder for the cardamom. Experiment and have fun!

Line an 8-by-8-in [20-by-20-cm] pan with parchment paper (see page 19). Set aside.

In a medium saucepan over medium heat, combine the cream, butter, **canna butter**, cardamom, and salt. Warm just until the butter melts (don't let it boil) about 4 minutes. Remove from the heat.

CONT'D

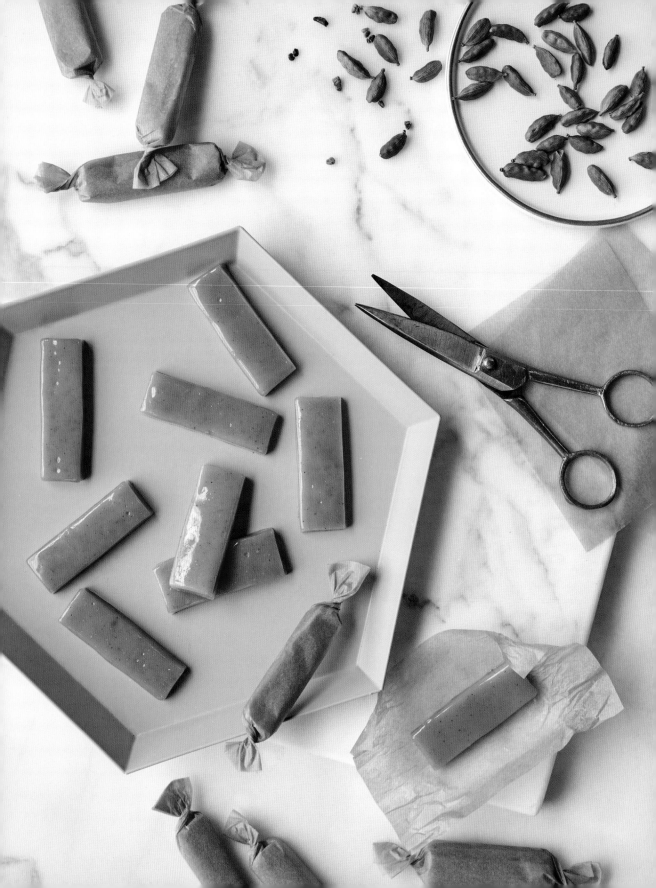

In a 3½-qt [3.3-L] saucepan (size matters because the caramel will bubble up) over medium-high heat, combine the corn syrup and water. (If using a candy thermometer, clip it to the saucepan.) Pour the sugar directly into the center of the liquids to avoid any sugar getting onto the sides of the pan. If you do get sugar on the sides, wash it down using a pastry brush dipped in water. Cook the sugar mixture, letting it come to a boil without stirring, for about 6 minutes. At about 250°F [120°C], the sugar syrup will start to boil rapidly. (If using an instant-read thermometer, check the temperature by tilting the pan so the probe measures the temperature of the syrup and not the bottom of the pan. The syrup will be bubbling aggressively, so be careful.) If there are any bits of sugar that have not melted yet, nudge them gently with the tip of your thermometer or a knife. Continue to cook for about 10 minutes more until the syrup reaches 320°F [160°C]. Because there is a small volume of syrup, you may need to tip the pan to get an accurate temperature reading. That's fine, but, otherwise, avoid any unnecessary stirring.

Once the syrup hits 320°F [160°C], gently stir it with a rubber spatula while slowly pouring the warm cream mixture into the sugar syrup. The liquid will bubble up and triple in size. Let the caramel return to a boil, stirring constantly to keep the bottom from burning. Cook for about 5 minutes until the caramel reaches 250°F [120°C]. When the caramel is close to temperature, stir in the vanilla bean paste.

Quickly pour the caramel into the prepared pan, scraping the bottom and sides with the rubber spatula. Let cool completely, at least 3 hours or, ideally, overnight. When the caramel has set, lift it out of the pan by the parchment.

Spray a sharp knife with baking spray. Working quickly, cut the caramel block into four equal quarters. Halve each quarter vertically, then, cutting horizontally, divide each half into six even pieces. Each caramel should measure 2 in by 1 in [5 cm by 2.5 cm]. If the caramels become too soft to handle, refrigerate them to firm up.

To wrap your caramels, cut forty-eight 3-by-4-in [7.5-by-10-cm] pieces of parchment paper, wax paper, or cellophane candy wrappers. Wrap each caramel in paper and crease it, then twist the ends closed. Store the wrapped caramels in an airtight container at room temperature for up to one week, or freeze for up to six months.

Booty Call Brownies

| ACTIVE TIME: **45 minutes** | INACTIVE TIME: **1 hour, 15 minutes** | MAKES: **18 3-by-2-in brownies** |

FUDGY BROWNIE

8 oz | 230 g unsalted butter

1½ cups plus 3 Tbsp | 345 g sugar

½ cup plus ⅓ cup | 98 g unsweetened Dutch-process cocoa powder (see Note, page 78)

1 tsp kosher salt

1 tsp vanilla extract

3 large eggs

¾ cup | 105 g all-purpose flour

COOKIE DOUGH SPREAD

1 cup | 140 g all-purpose flour

6 oz | 170 g unsalted butter, at room temperature

2¾ tsp | 12 g Canna Butter (page 27)

½ cup | 100 g sugar

1 cup | 200 g packed light brown sugar

CONT'D

We could not write an edibles cookbook without including a pot brownie, so here it is: the most over-the-top, indulgent, and irresistible brownie ever. We give you Booty Call Brownies—a fudgy masterpiece slathered with a chocolate chip cookie dough spread and crowned with chocolate sandwich cookies. Combining all these things into one ridiculously decadent, NSFW, come-hither brownie comes from a place of questionable judgment—it's so wrong, but feels oh so right. This is the kind of brownie that would do well on Tinder. Swipe right.

TO MAKE THE FUDGY BROWNIE: Preheat the oven to 325°F (165°C).

Line a 9-by-13-in [23-by-33-cm] pan with parchment paper (see page 19).

In a medium heatproof bowl over a double boiler, melt together the butter, sugar, cocoa powder, and salt. Cook for about 10 minutes, using a rubber spatula to stir the mixture occasionally until the butter melts and the batter starts to come together. It will look thick and grainy, and may even seem curdled. Don't worry. It will smooth out later.

Remove the bowl from the heat and let cool for 5 minutes. Stir in the vanilla. Transfer the batter to the bowl of a stand mixer fitted with the paddle attachment.

CONT'D

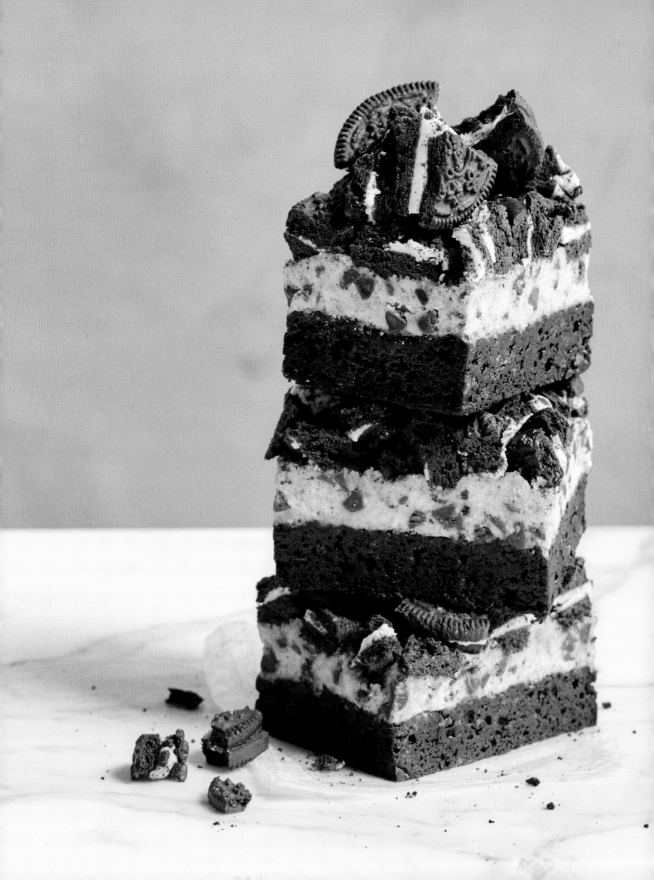

½ tsp kosher salt

2 Tbsp heavy cream or whole milk

1 tsp vanilla extract

¾ cup | 135 g mini chocolate chips

FINISHING TOUCHES
3½ cups | 250 g roughly chopped chocolate sandwich cookies

SPECIAL EQUIPMENT
Double boiler (page 19)

NOTE
Cocoa powders can vary in density, so, if possible, weighing this ingredient is best.

MAKE-AHEAD TIP
You can bake the brownies and toast the flour one day in advance. Cover the brownies with plastic wrap and refrigerate them. Store the flour in an airtight container at room temperature.

One egg at a time, beat in the eggs on low speed, waiting until one is incorporated before adding the next, 1 to 2 minutes. Scrape down the bowl with a rubber spatula about halfway through. When the batter looks shiny and smooth, add the flour. Mix for about 1 minute on low speed until it is incorporated and looks like the luscious, velvety, brownie batter of your dreams. Alternatively, mix everything the old-fashioned way with a wooden spoon and some elbow grease.

Pour the brownie batter into the prepared baking pan, scraping out the bowl with a rubber spatula. Bake for about 25 minutes until set. Let cool until you can touch the pan. Transfer to the refrigerator to cool faster.

TO MAKE THE COOKIE DOUGH SPREAD: Lower the oven temperature to 250°F (120°C). Line a rimmed baking sheet with parchment paper.

Spread the flour on the prepared sheet. Bake for 15 minutes, stirring halfway through the baking time. Let the toasted flour cool before using.

In the bowl of a stand mixer fitted with the paddle attachment, combine the butter, **canna butter**, sugar, brown sugar, and salt. Cream the mixture for about 2 minutes on medium speed until light and fluffy, pausing halfway through mixing to scrape down the sides of the bowl with a rubber spatula. Add the cream and vanilla and continue mixing until incorporated. Scrape down the sides of the bowl again with a rubber spatula. Adjust the speed to low, add the toasted flour, and mix for about 1 minute until it is evenly combined. Stir in the chocolate chips. Set aside at room temperature until the brownies have cooled.

TO ASSEMBLE: Using an offset spatula or pastry scraper, spread the cookie dough topping over the cooled brownies. Place a piece of plastic wrap over the cookie dough. Use your hands to press the dough into an even layer. Remove the plastic. Scatter the cookie pieces on top. Gently press them into the cookie dough spread.

Chill the brownies thoroughly (this is important to get clean cuts) for about 30 minutes before cutting. Run a knife along the sides of the brownie pan and use the parchment paper to lift the brownies out of the pan. Cut the brownies into eighteen 3-by-2-in (7.5-by-5-cm) pieces. Wipe your knife between cuts to keep the cuts sharp and clean.

These are best enjoyed right away (as if you could resist!). Refrigerate any leftovers in an airtight container for one to two days, or freeze for up to one month. Thaw at room temperature before serving.

Grapefruit Negroni *"Pot" de Fruits*

ACTIVE TIME: **45 minutes**	INACTIVE TIME: **3 hours**	MAKES: **64 pieces**

These jewel-like jelly candies, traditionally called *pâte de fruits* by French confectioners, are like the fancy, grownup version of fruit gummies. A fun play on the Negroni cocktail, we use Campari, sweet vermouth, and even infuse the rolling sugar in ground juniper berries to evoke the gin component. There are a few specialty ingredients involved, but the result is worth it. Sweet, tart, and slightly bitter, these brilliant bursts of flavor are a real showstopper. Put these beauties out as *mignardises* (French for fancy little after-dinner treats) and wait for the standing ovation.

GF | DF

3½ cups plus 1 tsp | 705 g sugar

2 Tbsp | 13 g apple pectin (see Note, page 81)

1½ tsp | 7 g tartaric acid or fresh lemon juice (see Note, page 81)

3½ tsp | 14 g water

2 cups | 500 g grapefruit juice (unstrained, not from concentrate)

½ cup | 120 g Campari

¼ cup | 60 g sweet vermouth

6 Tbsp plus 1½ tsp | 130 g light corn syrup

2 Tbsp plus 2 tsp | 32 g Canna Tincture (page 33)

1 Tbsp | 6 g dried juniper berries

½ cup | 100 g raw sugar

SPECIAL EQUIPMENT

Instant-read thermometer or candy thermometer

Coffee grinder or spice grinder

Spray an 8-by-8-in [20-by-20-cm] baking pan with nonstick baking spray.

Remove ⅓ cup plus 2 tsp [75 g] sugar from your total amount of sugar and place it in a small bowl with the pectin. Stir together until evenly mixed.

In another small bowl, dissolve the tartaric acid in the water.

In a large saucepan (at least 4-qt [3.8-L] as the mixture will bubble up a lot) over medium-high heat, stir together the grapefruit juice, Campari, and sweet vermouth. Bring to a boil, about 5 minutes.

CONT'D

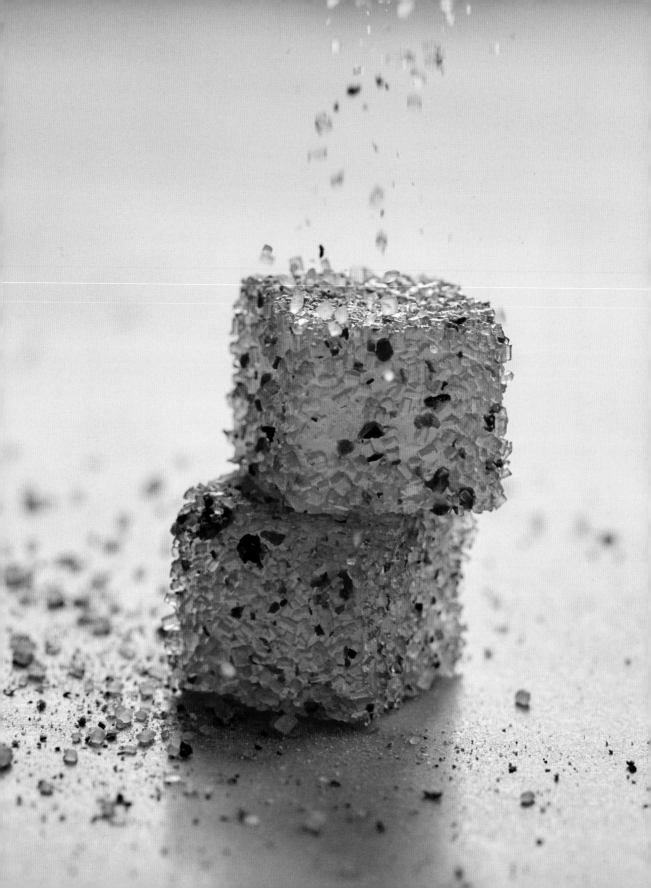

For this recipe, we use Solgar apple pectin powder.

Tartaric acid is often used in confections to impart a distinctive tartness. You can substitute fresh lemon juice for tartaric acid, but do not replace it with cream of tartar.

VARIATION

Play with the kind of sugar you use for rolling. We chose raw sugar for its flavor and appearance. Granulated sugar will give a finer mouthfeel. White sparkling sanding sugar lets more of the candy's color show through.

Slowly sprinkle in the pectin-sugar mixture, stirring constantly. Let the mixture come to a boil, and boil for 1 full minute. Add the remaining sugar and the corn syrup. (If using a candy thermometer, clip it to the saucepan.) Cook for 10 to 15 minutes until it reaches 220°F [104°C], stirring frequently with a rubber spatula to keep the bottom from burning. (If using an instant-read thermometer, check the temperature by tilting the pan so the probe measures the temperature of the syrup and not the bottom of the pan.) Add the **canna tincture**. Continue cooking for about 3 minutes more, to 224°F [107°C], stirring frequently. Remove from the heat.

Stir in the tartaric acid-water mixture and mix well. Working quickly and using a rubber spatula to scrape out the pot, transfer the candy to the prepared pan. Pop any air bubbles with a toothpick or the tip of a paring knife. Let sit at room temperature until completely cool and firm, about 3 hours, or up to overnight.

Meanwhile, make the sugar coating: In a clean coffee grinder, pulverize the juniper berries and 1 tsp raw sugar. Transfer to a large bowl and whisk in the remaining raw sugar until well combined. Set aside.

To unmold the candy, invert the pan over a cutting board. Coat a sharp knife with baking spray. Cut the candy into sixty-four 1-in [2.5-cm] squares. Drop them into the bowl of juniper-infused sugar and toss to coat.

Store in an airtight container at room temperature for up to one month. If the candies start to get sticky, re-sugar them in the juniper-infused sugar.

Blood Orange Shatter Blondies

| ACTIVE TIME: **35 minutes** | INACTIVE TIME: **45 minutes** | MAKES: **12 blondies** |

Rich and chewy, these brown butter blondies are studded with walnuts and show off beautiful blood oranges (quite possibly the sexiest citrus fruit around). Because we love to push things over the top (call us overachievers), we add a caramel shatter on top before baking. Besides simply looking rad—like brilliant shards of stained glass—the shatter melts into the batter as it bakes, effectively candying the orange slices and forming delicious toffee-like puddles throughout the blondies. One taste and you'll agree—this is A+ work here.

BLOOD ORANGE SHATTER

1 blood orange or navel orange if blood oranges are out of season

¾ cup | 150 g sugar

BLONDIES

8 oz | 230 g unsalted butter

2 tsp | 9 g Canna Butter (page 27)

2 large eggs

1½ cups | 300 g packed light brown sugar

1¾ cups | 245 g all-purpose flour

1¼ tsp baking powder

1½ tsp kosher salt

¾ cup | 90 g walnuts, roughly chopped

1 blood orange or navel orange if blood oranges are out of season, sliced into ⅛-in [3-mm] circles

TO MAKE THE BLOOD ORANGE SHATTER: Zest and juice the orange. Set the zest aside. In a medium saucepan over medium-low heat, combine 2 Tbsp orange juice and the sugar. Cook without disturbing (do not stir) for about 3 minutes until the sugar starts to dissolve. Raise the heat to medium-high and cook until the caramel is a deep golden brown-amber color, about 5 minutes more.

Meanwhile, line a baking sheet with a silicone baking mat or parchment paper and spray it with nonstick baking spray. Pour the caramel onto the prepared sheet pan in a thin even layer. Sprinkle the zest all over the shatter. Let cool completely. Peel the caramel off and transfer it to a cutting board. Using a sharp knife, break the hard caramel into small shards. Be careful, the edges can be sharp. Set the shatter aside while you prepare the blondie batter.

CONT'D

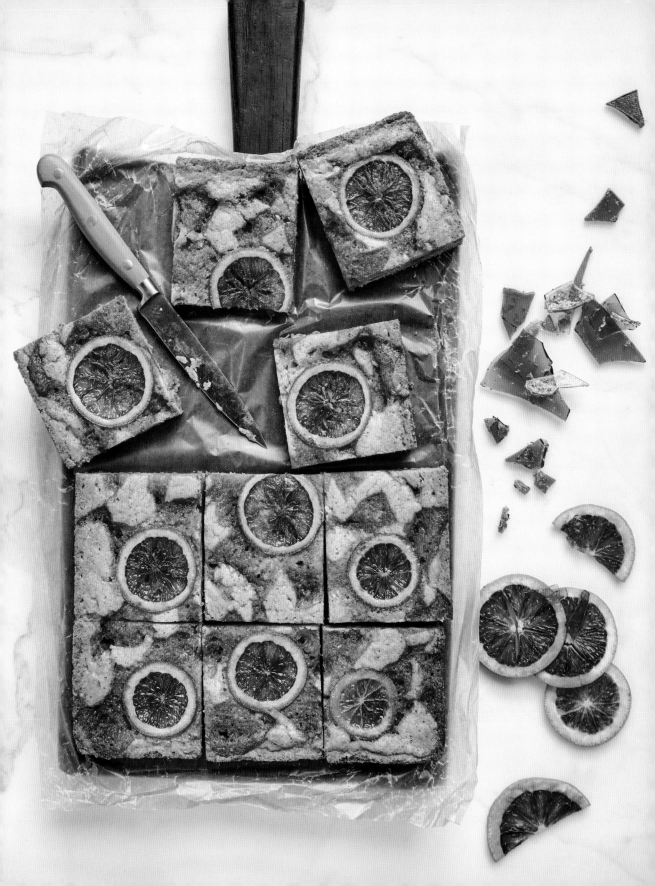

TO MAKE THE BLONDIES: Preheat the oven to 320°F [160°C].

Line a 9-by-13-in [23-by-33-cm] baking pan with parchment paper (see page 19).

In a small saucepan over medium heat, melt the unsalted butter slowly for 5 to 7 minutes until it turns golden brown. The butter will foam up and you will see golden flecks rise to the surface. Swirl it to see if the butter beneath the foam is turning golden. It will smell fragrant, nutty, and heavenly. If you're unsure about whether it's done, pour the butter into a glass measuring cup. If it isn't browned yet, pour it back into the pan to cook longer. Don't get distracted: the butter can go from golden brown to burnt quickly. Once your butter is browned, pour it into a measuring cup or small bowl (discard any burnt bits stuck to the bottom of the pan; they'll be bitter). Add the **canna butter** and let it melt. Set aside to cool for about 15 minutes.

In a large bowl, whisk the eggs and brown sugar until frothy. Whisk in the butter mixture. In a separate large bowl, whisk the flour, baking powder, and salt. Fold the flour mixture and walnuts into the wet ingredients until just combined. Pour the batter into the prepared baking pan and smooth the top with a rubber spatula. Arrange the orange slices on top of the batter, lightly pushing them down. Scatter all the caramel shatter on top. Bake for 30 to 35 minutes until the top is golden and set. The center will still be a little gooey.

Let the blondies cool completely in the pan. Lift them out using the parchment and cut them into twelve equal 3-by-3¼-in [7.5-by-8-cm] pieces.

Store in an airtight container for up to three days at room temperature, or freeze for up to six months. Thaw at room temperature before serving.

Frozen Key Lime Pies

| ACTIVE TIME: **40 minutes** | INACTIVE TIME: **4 hours** | MAKES: **12 mini pies** |

Sweet and tart, cool and refreshing, with a texture like soft ice cream, these mini frozen key lime pies are perfect for summer entertaining. We love that they can be made in advance, so you can focus on being the fabulous host you are. The single-serving size is convenient as well. You won't have to split a dose . . . which means you won't have to share your personal pie (you're welcome).

GRAHAM CRACKER CRUST

½ cup plus 1 Tbsp | 65 g graham cracker crumbs (from 4 to 5 whole graham crackers)

¼ cup | 50 g sugar

6 Tbsp | 85 g unsalted butter, melted

2 tsp | 9 g Canna Butter (page 27), melted

KEY LIME FILLING

7 medium limes

6 large egg yolks | 120 g, at room temperature

¼ cup | 50 g sugar

One 14-oz | 400-g can sweetened condensed milk

CONT'D

TO MAKE THE GRAHAM CRACKER CRUST: Preheat the oven to 350°F [180°C]. Line a 12-cup muffin pan with cupcake liners and set aside.

In a food processor, blitz together the graham cracker crumbs and sugar until combined. Add the butter and **canna butter** and process until evenly distributed. Fill each cup with an equal amount of the graham crust mixture, about 2 Tbsp plus 1 tsp [17 g]. For the most accurate dosage, weigh the total amount of the crust mixture and divide by twelve to determine the target weight per serving. Press the crumbs down using the bottom of a shot glass to create an even bottom crust. Don't worry about getting the crust up the sides. Bake for about 10 minutes until golden. Remove from the oven and cool completely.

TO MAKE THE KEY LIME FILLING: While the crusts cool, zest and juice 6 of the limes. You will need 2 Tbsp packed lime zest and ¾ cup [175 g] lime juice. Reserve any extra zest for garnishing.

CONT'D

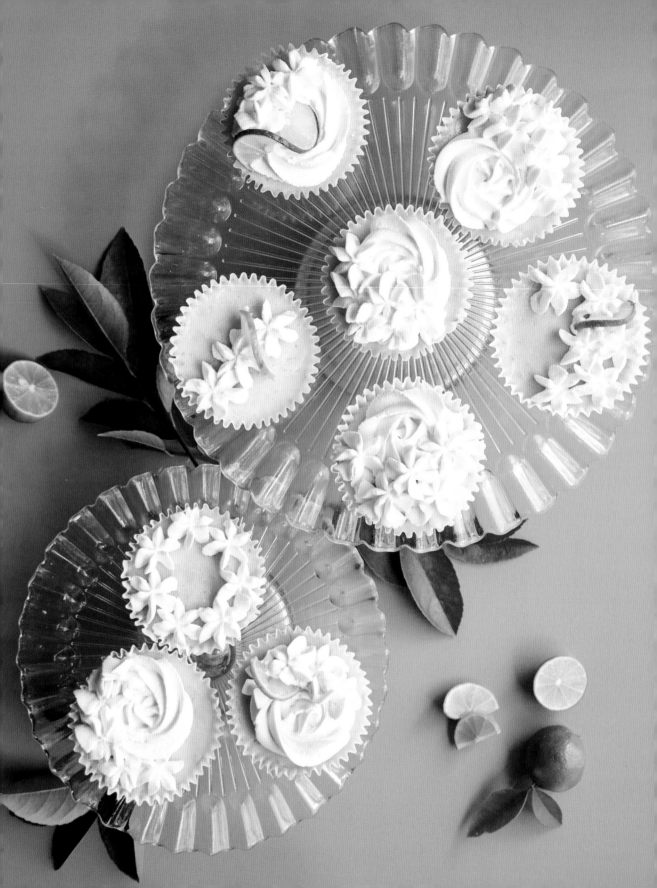

1 pt | 460 g heavy cream, cold

2 Tbsp powdered sugar

1 tsp vanilla extract

12-cup muffin pan

Shot glass

Pastry bag and star tip
(optional)

The pies can be made up to three
days in advance. Prepare them up
to the whipped cream step, cover
the muffin tin tightly with plastic
wrap, and keep frozen until ready
to serve.

Fill a medium saucepan with 1 to 2 in [3 to 5 cm] of water and bring it
to barely a simmer over medium-high heat. Adjust the heat to low.

In a medium heatproof bowl, whisk the egg yolks, lime juice, and
sugar until combined. Set the bowl over the saucepan (the bottom
of the bowl shouldn't touch the surface of the water), and cook for
about 5 minutes, whisking constantly, until the mixture is frothy and
puddinglike.

Remove the bowl from the heat. Whisk in the sweetened condensed
milk and lime zest until well combined. Divide the filling equally among
the 12 cups, about $\frac{1}{3}$ cup of filling per portion.

Freeze until firm, at least 4 hours.

WHEN READY TO SERVE, MAKE THE WHIPPED CREAM: In a
large bowl, combine the cream, powdered sugar, and vanilla. Using
a handheld electric mixer, beat for about 1 minute on high speed
until medium to stiff peaks form. Alternatively, you can whisk by hand
(earn that whipped cream!) or use a stand mixer. Dollop the cream
on top of each pie, or, if you're feeling fancy, transfer it to a pastry bag
fitted with a star tip and pipe decoratively.

Cut the remaining lime into thin slices and garnish the pies, along
with any extra lime zest. Enjoy immediately.

Black Sesame & Raspberry Cupcakes

| ACTIVE TIME: **1 hour** | INACTIVE TIME: **0 minutes** | MAKES: **24 mini cupcakes** |

½ cup plus 2 Tbsp | 90 g black sesame seeds

BLACK SESAME CUPCAKES

½ cup plus 2 Tbsp | 70 g cake flour (see Note, page 91)

½ tsp baking powder

Pinch of baking soda

Pinch of kosher salt

1 Tbsp | 14 g unsalted butter, at room temperature

1 Tbsp plus 1¼ tsp | 18 g Canna Butter (page 27), at room temperature

¼ cup | 50 g granulated sugar

2 large egg whites

CONT'D

Unexpected, chic, and oh so delicious, these are not your run-of-the-mill, ho-hum cupcakes. You definitely won't be seeing them at any neighborhood bake sale. (If you do, give them all your money!) At first glance these look like they could be chocolate cupcakes with a cookies 'n' cream frosting. We love that they're not. Rich in flavor, sweet and fragrant, toasty and nutty, black sesame is about to have its moment—we're calling it now. The frosting alone is so good you'll be licking the beaters clean. And that hidden raspberry treasure tucked inside? Well, now, that takes the (cup)cake.

Preheat the oven to 350°F [180°C]. Coat a mini muffin pan with nonstick baking spray or cupcake liners and set aside.

In a dry skillet over medium heat, spread the sesame seeds and toast for about 5 minutes until fragrant. Working in batches, transfer to a clean coffee grinder or spice grinder. Grind the seeds to the texture of sand. Set aside 6 Tbsp [55 g] of the ground sesame seeds for the buttercream frosting.

TO MAKE THE BLACK SESAME CUPCAKES: In a large bowl, whisk ¼ cup [35 g] of the ground sesame seeds, the cake flour, baking powder, baking soda, and salt until well combined.

CONT'D

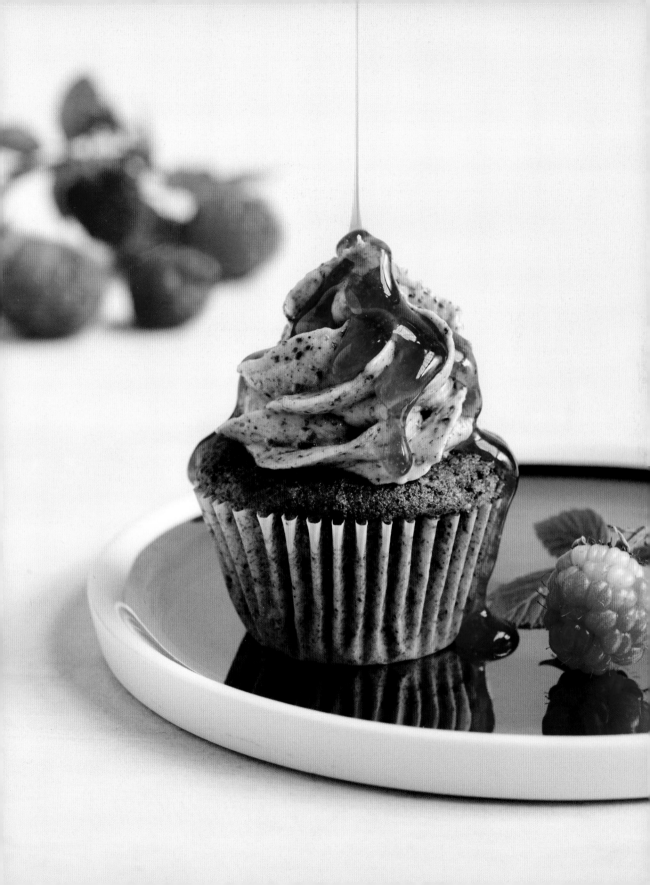

1 tsp vanilla extract

¼ cup plus 1 Tbsp | 75 g
full-fat sour cream

¼ cup | 60 g whole milk

24 whole raspberries
(about ½ pt | 120 g)

RASPBERRY COULIS

2 cups | 240 g fresh
raspberries

BLACK SESAME
BUTTERCREAM

8 oz | 230 g unsalted butter,
at room temperature

2 cups | 240 g powdered
sugar

1 tsp vanilla extract

¾ tsp toasted sesame oil

½ tsp kosher salt

SPECIAL EQUIPMENT

24-cup mini muffin pan

Coffee grinder or spice
grinder

Fine-mesh strainer

Pastry bag and decorative tip
(optional)

Using a handheld electric mixer, or in the bowl of a stand mixer fitted with a paddle attachment, beat the butter and **canna butter** for about 1 minute on high speed until smooth and creamy. Add the sugar. Beat for about 2 minutes on high speed until the mixture is creamed together, light, and fluffy, pausing to scrape down the bowl with a rubber spatula.

Add the egg whites and vanilla. Beat for about 1 minute on medium-high speed just until well combined. Beat in the sour cream until combined. Scrape down the bowl again.

Turn the mixer to low speed, add the dry ingredients, and mix until just incorporated. With the mixer still on low speed, slowly pour in the milk and mix until just combined. Do not overmix. Scrape down the bowl, making sure there are no lumps at the bottom of the bowl.

Equally distribute the batter among the 24 prepared mini muffin cups. Each should be about two-thirds full, containing about 1 Tbsp [22 g] of batter. For the most accurate dosage, weigh the total amount of batter and divide by twenty-four to determine the target weight per serving. Push one whole raspberry, open-side down, into each cup to submerge it. The tip of the raspberry should just hit the surface.

Bake for 11 to 13 minutes until firm, spongy, and slightly golden at the edges, or until a toothpick inserted in the center comes out clean, rotating the pan halfway through the baking time. Let cool completely on a wire rack.

TO MAKE THE RASPBERRY COULIS: While the cupcakes bake, toss the raspberries in a blender for about 2 minutes until very smooth, scraping down the sides of the blender as needed. Strain the purée through a fine-mesh strainer to get a smooth, seedless sauce. Transfer to a condiment squeeze bottle or glass jar. Cover and refrigerate until ready to use, or for up to one week.

If you don't have cake flour, you can make your own. To make 1 cup [140 g] of cake flour, measure 1 cup [140 g] of all-purpose flour. Remove 2 Tbsp [20 g] of flour and replace with 2 Tbsp [20 g] cornstarch. Sift together the flour and cornstarch three to four times to incorporate and aerate it.

MAKE-AHEAD TIP

The cupcakes can be made ahead and kept in an airtight container at room temperature for up to one day. The frosting can be made ahead and kept in an airtight container at room temperature for up to three days. If leaving butter out at room temperature gives you the willies, refrigerate it, but allow time for it to come back to room temperature before you attempt to pipe it. You may need to paddle it in the mixer again to soften it to an easily spreadable texture.

The raspberry coulis can be made ahead and refrigerated in an airtight container for up to one week. If transporting the cupcakes, reserve the raspberry coulis and drizzle it on right before serving.

TO MAKE THE BLACK SESAME BUTTERCREAM: In the bowl of a stand mixer fitted with the paddle attachment, or in a large bowl with a handheld mixer, combine the buttercream ingredients and the remaining 6 Tbsp [55 g] of ground toasted sesame seeds. Mix on low speed until the powdered sugar is incorporated. Raise the speed to medium-high and mix for 1 to 2 minutes until the buttercream is fluffy and evenly combined, pausing to scrape down the sides of the bowl a few times.

If you wish, transfer the frosting to a pastry bag fitted with a decorative tip (we're fans of the Wilton 1M tip for this), or a resealable plastic bag with a bottom corner snipped off. Alternatively, use an offset spatula or butter knife to spread the buttercream. Decorate each cupcake with buttercream and add a drizzle of raspberry coulis. Enjoy immediately.

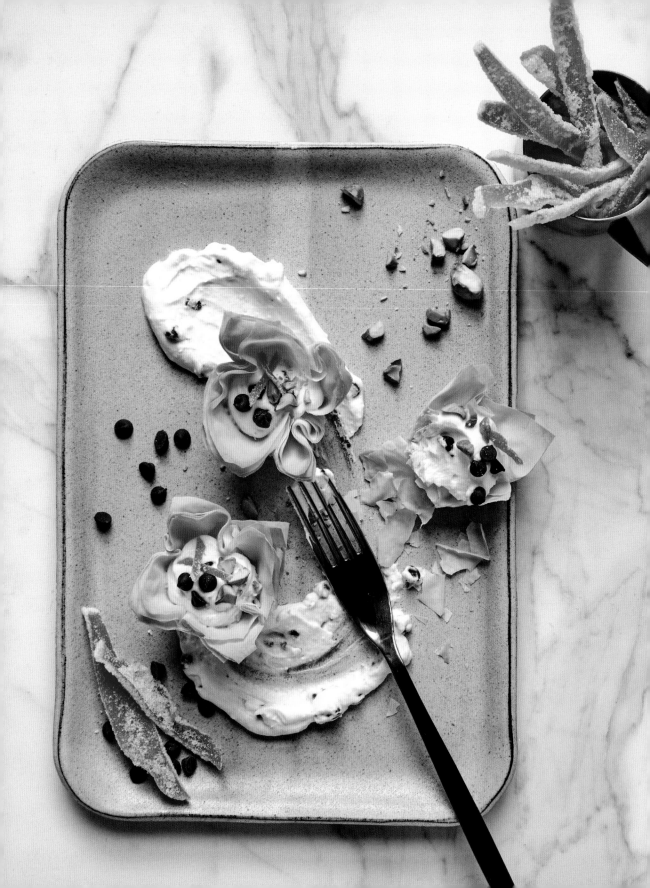

Cannoli Cups

ACTIVE TIME: **45 minutes** INACTIVE TIME: **0 minutes** MAKES: **24 mini cups**

PHYLLO CUPS

One 1-lb | 455-g package frozen phyllo dough, thawed in the refrigerator

CANNOLI CREAM

1 cup | 240 g high-quality whole-milk ricotta cheese, drained of excess liquid (see Note, page 94)

¼ cup | 60 g mascarpone cheese

2 Tbsp powdered sugar

1 Tbsp plus 1½ tsp | 19 g Canna Coconut Oil (page 29)

½ tsp vanilla extract

¼ tsp kosher salt

¼ cup | 45 g mini chocolate chips, plus more for garnishing

FINISHING TOUCHES

¼ cup | 35 g raw pistachios, finely chopped

Candied orange peel, cut into thin 1-in [2.5-cm] long strips, for garnishing

SPECIAL EQUIPMENT

24-cup mini muffin pan

Victoria Pastry Company in North Beach, the Little Italy of San Francisco, California, has been making the best cannoli in the city for more than one hundred years. Simple, classic, perfect, those cannoli are the inspiration behind these mini cannoli cups. We employ ready-made phyllo dough to create a light, crisp shell, and ate so many of Victoria Pastry's cannoli to reverse engineer that heavenly cream filling (we know, pure dedication here). Pass around these classy little bites at your next party and get ready for the oohs and aahs.

Preheat the oven to 375°F (190°C). Spray a mini muffin pan with nonstick baking spray.

TO MAKE THE PHYLLO CUPS: Unroll the phyllo dough sheets onto a baking sheet and cover them with a piece of wax paper. Put a kitchen towel on top of the wax paper to weigh it down and protect it from the air. Phyllo dough is superthin and dries out very quickly if left uncovered.

Place one sheet of phyllo dough on a large cutting board, leaving the rest covered, and carefully spray it with butter or coconut oil baking spray. Place another sheet on top and spray it. Repeat until you have five sheets of dough stacked and sprayed. Don't forget to spray the top of the final layer. Roll up the leftover sheets of phyllo dough and refrigerate. Use within 2 days.

CONT'D

Since the ricotta is the star of the show, you can really taste the difference if you use a high-quality brand. We love Bellwether Farms' whole-milk basket ricotta made from pure Jersey cow's milk. It's insanely good. You may be ruined for life after tasting it.

MAKE-AHEAD TIP

The phyllo cups can be made ahead and stored in an airtight container at room temperature for up to one week, or frozen for up to one month. The filling can be made ahead and refrigerated in an airtight container for one day.

VARIATION

For a stronger dose, add a drizzle of Canna Honey (page 34) on top.

Cut the stack into 24 even rectangles: Divide the long side into six pieces and the short side into four pieces. Pick up one rectangle (pick up all the layers) and gently push the center into one of the muffin tin cups. Press the sides against the inside wall of the muffin mold to make sure a cup is formed. Repeat, forming 24 cups. Bake for 8 to 10 minutes until golden. Gently lift the phyllo cups out and place them onto a wire cooling rack. Cool the cups completely before filling.

TO MAKE THE CANNOLI CREAM: While the cups cool, in the bowl of a stand mixer fitted with the paddle attachment, combine the ricotta, mascarpone, powdered sugar, **canna coconut oil**, vanilla, and salt. Beat for about 3 minutes on medium speed until smooth and evenly combined, pausing about halfway through the mixing to scrape down the sides of the bowl with a rubber spatula. (Alternatively, use a handheld electric mixer.) Stir in the chocolate chips. For the most accurate dosage, weigh the total amount of cannoli cream and divide by twenty-four to determine the amount of filling per cup. Transfer the filling to a piping bag or resealable plastic bag with one corner snipped off.

Place a phyllo cup on the scale, tare the weight, and then pipe until you reach the target weight (about 16 g). Alternatively, equally divide the cannoli cream among the phyllo cups, filling them to the rim. Garnish each cannoli cup with a sprinkling of chocolate chips and pistachios, and top with candied orange peel. Enjoy immediately.

Duck Meatball Sliders

| ACTIVE TIME: **40 minutes** | INACTIVE TIME: **0 minutes** | MAKES: **12 sliders** |

Sweet, savory, and kissed with a balance of warm spices, these sliders are not your typical game-day sliders. Because remember when you made your own duck meatballs from scratch? Yeah, that was boss.

SPICED PLUM CHUTNEY

²/₃ cup plus 2 Tbsp | 240 g plum chutney or jam

2 tsp | 8 g Canna Butter (page 27)

1 tsp Chinese five-spice powder

½ tsp granulated onion

HERBED AIOLI

1 garlic clove, minced

Pinch of kosher salt, plus more as needed

½ cup | 120 g mayonnaise

1 tsp finely chopped fresh flat-leaf parsley

1 tsp finely chopped fresh cilantro

DUCK MEATBALLS

1 lb | 455 g boneless duck breast (2 to 3 breasts; skin left on one breast), cut into 2-in [5-cm] pieces

CONT'D

TO MAKE THE SPICED PLUM CHUTNEY: In a small saucepan over medium heat, warm the plum chutney for about 3 minutes. Remove from the heat. Whisk in the **canna butter**, Chinese five-spice powder, and granulated onion until the butter is well incorporated and evenly distributed. Set aside.

TO MAKE THE HERBED AIOLI: On a cutting board, combine the minced garlic and a pinch of salt. Using the side of your chef's knife, press it into the cutting board and mash the garlic into a paste. Transfer to a small bowl and add the mayonnaise. Whisk to combine. Add the parsley and cilantro and whisk to combine. Taste and season with more salt, if needed. Transfer to an airtight container and refrigerate until ready to use.

TO MAKE THE DUCK MEATBALLS: Preheat the oven to 350°F [180°C]. Line a rimmed sheet pan with parchment paper and set aside.

Add the duck to a food processor and pulse about 15 times, stopping a few times to scrape down the sides with a rubber spatula, until you have an evenly ground-up mixture.

CONT'D

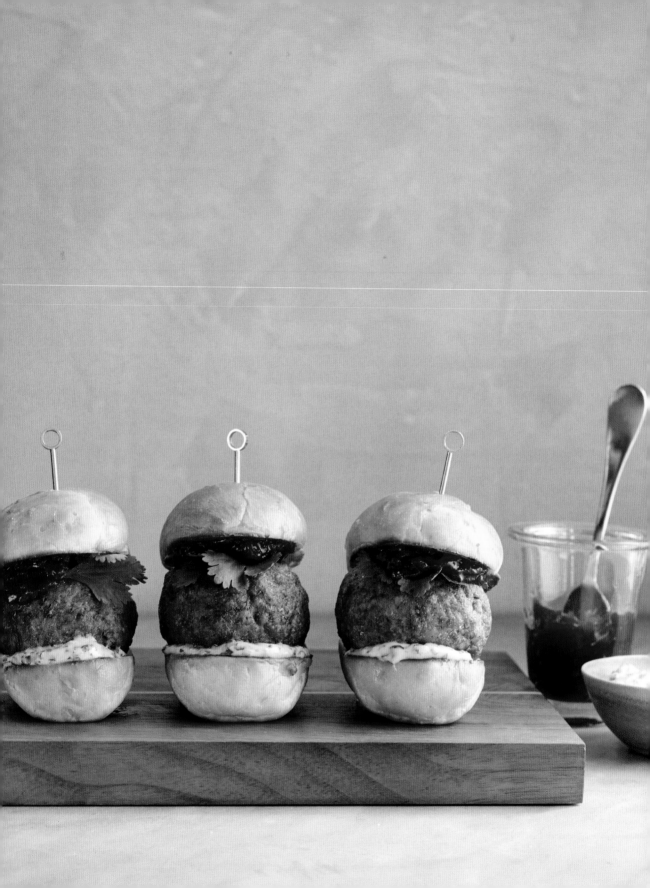

1 lb | 455 g ground pork

1 large egg

½ cup | 30 g panko bread crumbs

2 Tbsp finely chopped scallion

1 Tbsp plus 1 tsp soy sauce

1 Tbsp Chinese five-spice powder

1 Tbsp kosher salt, plus more for seasoning

1 tsp freshly ground black pepper, plus more for seasoning

1 Tbsp grapeseed oil or vegetable oil

TO ASSEMBLE

12 Hawaiian sweet rolls or slider rolls

Unsalted butter, at room temperature

Kosher salt

Freshly ground black pepper

MAKE-AHEAD TIP

The meatball mixture can be made one day ahead and refrigerated in an airtight container. Or, form the meatballs, freeze, and keep frozen in an airtight container for up to one month. Defrost them in the refrigerator overnight before cooking.

VARIATION

For a stronger dose, use the Gruyère & Green Garlic Gougères (page 98) as your buns. Be prepared never to want to eat a slider any other way again.

In the bowl of a stand mixer fitted with the paddle attachment, combine the ground duck, pork, egg, bread crumbs, scallion, soy sauce, Chinese five-spice powder, salt, and pepper. Mix for 1 to 2 minutes on low speed until all ingredients are well combined. Divide the mixture into 12 portions and roll each into a meatball.

In a large skillet or sauté pan over medium-high heat, heat the oil. Working in batches so you don't crowd the pan, add the meatballs to sear, turning every minute or so until you get a nice crust all around. Transfer to the prepared sheet pan. Place the pan in the oven and cook for 10 to 15 minutes until the meatballs are firm to the touch and cooked through to an internal temperature of 165°F [74°C]. Remove from the oven and turn on the broiler.

TO ASSEMBLE: Butter the cut sides of the rolls and season them with salt and pepper. Place them cut-side up on a sheet pan. Broil for 2 to 3 minutes until toasty, watching closely so they don't burn.

Spread 2 tsp herbed aioli on the bottom half of each roll. Place a meatball on top and finish with about 1 Tbsp [20 g] plum chutney and the roll top. For the most accurate dosage, weigh the total amount of medicated chutney and divide by twelve to determine the target weight per serving. Devour immediately.

Gruyère & Green Garlic Gougères

| ACTIVE TIME: **25 minutes** | INACTIVE TIME: **35 minutes** | MAKES: **14 gougères** |

3½ oz | 100 g unsalted butter

2½ tsp | 11 g Canna Butter (page 27)

1 cup | 237 g water

½ tsp kosher salt

¼ tsp sugar

¼ tsp freshly ground black pepper

1 cup | 140 g all-purpose flour

4 large eggs

4 oz | 115 g Gruyère cheese, finely shredded

1 Tbsp minced green garlic or scallions

SPECIAL EQUIPMENT
One 3-Tbsp [45-ml] cookie scoop

When green garlic appears in the markets, we know it's time to celebrate the coming of spring by whipping up a batch of these gougères. Plus, there is no better party trick than presenting your guests with a basket of warm cheese puffs, and watching them disappear like magic. You can also turn gougères into fancy sandwiches, serve them next to a charcuterie spread for a little DIY station, or, if you really want to go to the next level, serve the delectable Duck Meatball Sliders (page 95) in gougère buns.

Preheat the oven to 400°F [200°C]. Line 2 baking sheets with parchment paper or silicone baking mats and set aside.

In a medium saucepan over medium heat, combine the butter, **canna butter**, water, salt, sugar, and pepper. Bring to a boil.

Once the butter melts, add the flour all at once. With a wooden spoon (preferably a flat-edged one), begin stirring immediately until the mixture forms a ball and comes away from the sides of the pan. Continue to cook, stirring, until the mixture starts to look gritty on the bottom of the pan. The dryer the mixture becomes, the better it will absorb the eggs, and the puffier the gougères get in the oven. Transfer the dough to the bowl of a stand mixer fitted with the paddle attachment and beat the dough on medium-low speed for about 1 minute until it is just warm to the touch.

CONT'D

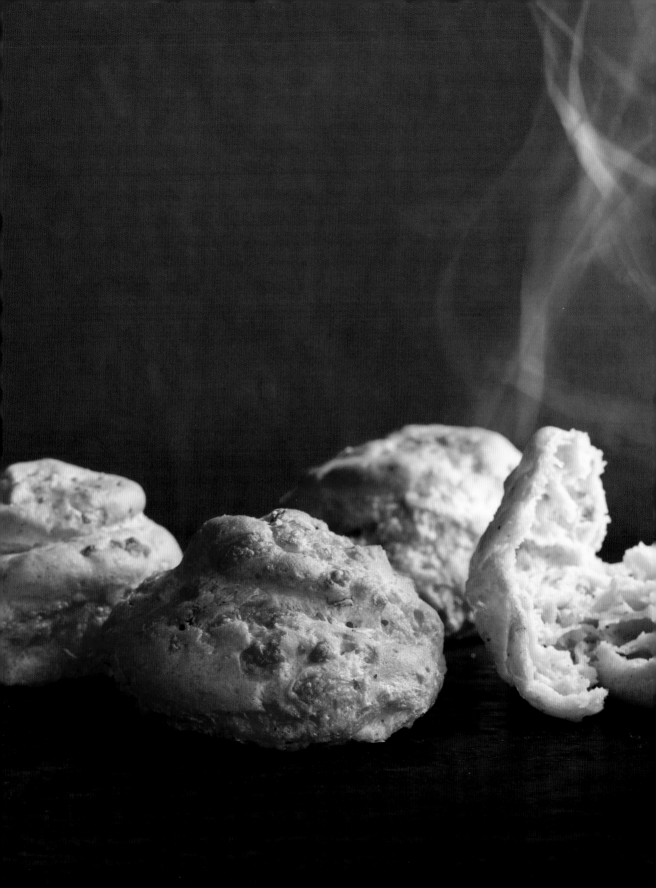

Increase the speed to medium-high and add the eggs one at a time, making sure each egg is fully incorporated into the batter before adding the next. At first, the egg will separate from the batter and it may seem as though it will never combine—but just as you start to lose hope it will magically come together to form a smooth, creamy, elastic batter. Scrape down the sides of the bowl between additions with a rubber spatula. Mix in the cheese and green garlic.

Coat a 3-Tbsp [45-ml] cookie scoop with nonstick baking spray and spoon out 7 level scoops of dough onto one of the prepared sheets, spacing them about 3 in [7.5 cm] apart. Respray the cookie scoop as needed. Spoon out 7 level scoops of dough onto the second prepared sheet, spacing them about 3 in [7.5 cm] apart. Wet your finger with a bit of water and smooth any jagged edges.

Bake for 30 to 35 minutes until the gougères are puffed, browned, and firm to the touch, rotating the sheets between racks and from front to back every 10 minutes. Keep an eye on them the last 5 minutes so they don't burn. They should sound hollow when tapped with your finger. Once done, cut a small slit in the side of each puff. Turn off the oven and return the gougères to the turned-off oven for 10 minutes to get extra crispy.

Transfer the baking sheets to a cooling rack. Enjoy while warm—there's nothing like a warm gougère fresh from the oven!

Refrigerate leftovers in an airtight container for up to three days, or freeze for up to three months. Re-crisp in a 400°F [200°C] oven for 2 to 3 minutes before serving.

Corn Dog Muffins

| ACTIVE TIME: **45 minutes** | INACTIVE TIME: **0 minutes** | MAKES: **24 mini muffins** |

This playful take on the corn dog is our version of a savory cupcake. Full of sweet corn and hot dogs, you'll feel like you're at the county fair. This portable little snack is the perfect thing to pack for a day at the park or an impromptu picnic. And don't forget that honey mustard spread! It really completes these bites, and leftovers make a perfect pretzel dip if you get a case of the munchies afterward.

GF

CORN DOG MUFFINS

2 Tbsp full-fat sour cream

2 Tbsp olive oil

1 Tbsp plus 2 tsp | 22 g Canna Coconut Oil (page 29)

1 large egg

¼ cup | 50 g granulated sugar

½ cup | 128 g canned cream-style sweet corn

½ cup | 75 g fine cornmeal

¼ cup | 35 g white rice flour

1 tsp baking powder

½ tsp kosher salt

3 beef hot dogs, cooked, each cut into 8 pieces

CONT'D

TO MAKE THE CORN DOG MUFFINS: Preheat the oven to 325°F [165°C]. Coat a mini muffin pan with nonstick baking spray and set aside.

In a medium bowl, combine the sour cream, olive oil, and **canna coconut oil**. Whisk until well combined and emulsified. Add the egg and sugar, and whisk again until well combined. Add the creamed corn and mix until just combined.

In a small bowl, whisk the cornmeal, rice flour, baking powder, and salt. Add the flour mixture to the corn mixture and whisk until just combined.

Equally distribute the batter among the 24 cups of the prepared mini muffin pan, filling each about two-thirds full (about 1 heaping Tbsp [18 g]). For the most accurate dosage, weigh the total amount of batter and divide by twenty-four to determine the target weight per serving. Press one hot dog slice into each cup, submerging it until the top hits the surface of the batter.

CONT'D

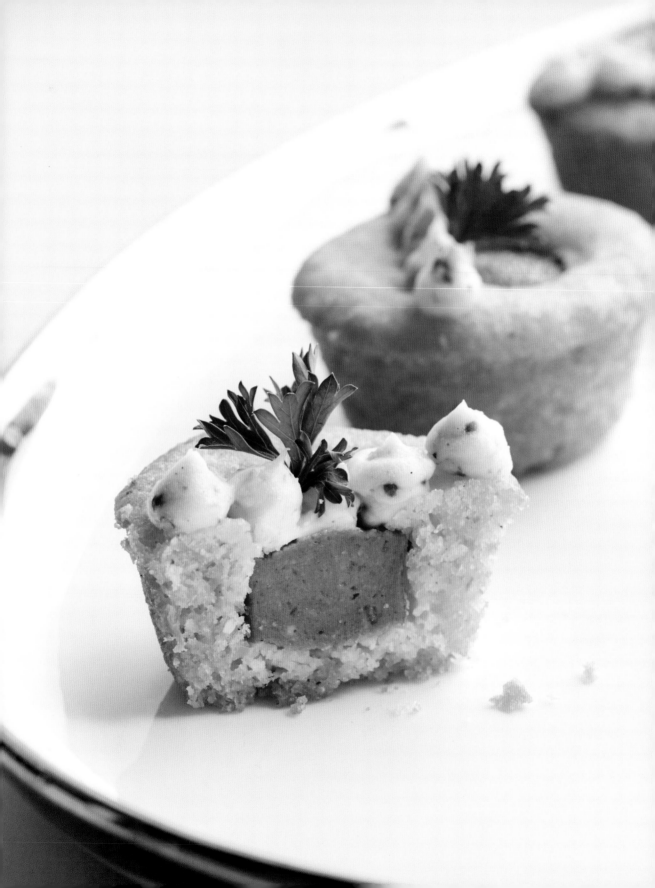

4 oz | 115 g cream cheese,
at room temperature

4 oz | 115 g unsalted butter,
at room temperature

1 Tbsp honey

2 Tbsp whole-grain
Dijon mustard

¾ tsp kosher salt

½ tsp freshly ground
black pepper, plus more
for seasoning

FINISHING TOUCHES

Flaky sea salt (see Note)

Freshly ground black pepper

Fresh parsley leaves
for garnishing

SPECIAL EQUIPMENT

24-cup mini muffin pan

NOTE

We use Maldon sea salt whenever
a recipe calls for flaky sea salt.
The large, crunchy flakes of salt
are perfect for final garnishes.

Bake for 25 to 27 minutes until golden brown (like a corn dog), or until a toothpick inserted in the muffin comes out clean. Remove the pan from the oven and cool for 5 minutes.

Invert the pan over a wire cooling rack to remove the muffins. Use a knife to help pop them out if needed. Let the muffins cool completely.

TO MAKE THE HONEY MUSTARD BUTTER: In the bowl of a stand mixer fitted with the paddle attachment, or using a bowl and a hand-held mixer, combine the cream cheese, butter, and honey. Beat for 1 to 2 minutes on medium speed until light and fluffy, scraping down the sides of the bowl with a rubber spatula once or twice. Add the mustard, salt, and pepper. Continue to beat on medium speed until well combined.

Dollop about 1 tsp of honey mustard butter onto each corn dog muffin. Finish with a touch of flaky sea salt and freshly ground black pepper. Garnish with parsley leaves. Transfer any remaining honey mustard butter to an airtight container and refrigerate for up to three days.

Cherry Cheesecakes

| ACTIVE TIME: **40 minutes** | INACTIVE TIME: **6 hours** | MAKES: **24 mini cheesecakes** |

GF

ALMOND BUCKWHEAT CRUST

2 Tbsp unsalted butter

1 Tbsp plus 2 tsp | 21 g Canna Butter (page 27)

½ cup | 60 g finely ground almond meal or almond flour

2 Tbsp buckwheat flour

2 Tbsp sugar

Pinch of kosher salt

Zest of ½ lemon

CHEESECAKE FILLING

½ cup | 115 g heavy cream

One 8-oz package | 230 g cream cheese, at room temperature

6 Tbsp | 60 g powdered sugar

1 tsp freshly squeezed lemon juice

½ tsp vanilla extract

CONT'D

A good make-ahead dessert can make entertaining seem effortless. These beautiful mini cheesecakes fill the bill. And the crust is so good, we don't blame you if you just want to eat it on its own like a cookie. Made with almond meal and buckwheat flour (a pseudo-cereal seed which, despite its name, is not related to wheat at all), this crust is gluten free and insanely delicious.

TO MAKE THE ALMOND BUCKWHEAT CRUST: Preheat the oven to 350°F [180°C]. Line a mini muffin pan with 24 mini cupcake liners.

In a small saucepan over medium heat, melt the unsalted butter. Alternatively, place it in a microwave-safe container and microwave for 30 seconds on high power just until melted. Remove from the heat and stir in the **canna butter** until melted together. Set aside to cool slightly.

In a medium bowl, stir together the almond flour, buckwheat flour, sugar, salt, and lemon zest. Stir in the melted butters and mix thoroughly to combine. Divide the crust equally among the muffin cups, filling each with about 1 packed tsp [6 g] of the mixture. For the most accurate dosage, weigh the total amount of the crust mixture and divide by twenty-four to determine the target weight per serving. Lightly press the mixture down using the bottom of a shot glass.

CONT'D

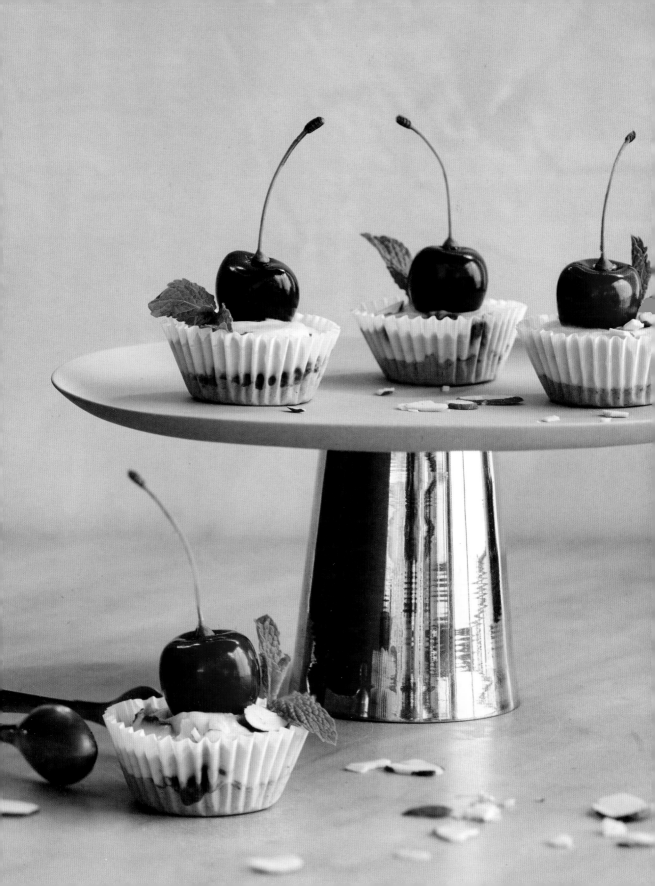

¼ tsp kosher salt

¾ cup | 100 g fresh or
½ cup | 100 g frozen cherries,
defrosted and drained, pitted
and roughly chopped

FINISHING TOUCHES
Fresh whole cherries

Toasted sliced almonds

Fresh mint leaves

SPECIAL EQUIPMENT
24-cup mini muffin pan

Shot glass

Pastry bag (optional)

MAKE-AHEAD TIP
These cheesecakes can be made ahead and kept refrigerated, covered with plastic wrap, for up to two days, or frozen for up to one month. If frozen, thaw in the refrigerator for 1 to 2 hours before serving.

Bake the crusts for about 10 minutes until lightly browned. Remove from the oven and cool for at least 10 minutes while preparing the filling.

TO MAKE THE CHEESECAKE FILLING: In the bowl of a stand mixer fitted with the whisk attachment, beat the cream for 2 to 3 minutes on medium-high speed until medium-soft peaks form. Alternatively, use a handheld mixer. Transfer the whipped cream to a medium bowl and set aside. Return the bowl to the mixer and swap the whisk for the paddle attachment.

In the stand mixer bowl, combine the cream cheese, powdered sugar, lemon juice, vanilla, and salt. Beat for 3 to 5 minutes on medium-high speed until smooth and creamy, pausing to scrape down the sides of the bowl with a rubber spatula, as needed. Alternatively, use a handheld electric mixer; it will take longer to achieve a smooth consistency. Scrape down the bowl and the paddle, and switch back to the whisk attachment.

Add the whipped cream to the bowl and mix for about 2 minutes on medium-high speed until the mixture holds stiff peaks.

Add the cherries and mix on medium speed just until the cherries begin to break apart. Using a rubber spatula, scrape down the bowl once again and fold the mixture a few times. Don't stress over getting it perfectly combined; some streaks are fine. Transfer the filling to a pastry bag or resealable plastic bag with a corner snipped off to about a ¾-in [2-cm] opening. Alternatively, fill the cups with a spoon, but we find piping is the easiest and cleanest way to fill the cups. Divide the filling equally among the crusts. Cover with plastic wrap and refrigerate for at least six hours, or ideally overnight, until the filling sets.

Before serving, decorate each cheesecake with a fresh cherry on top, a sprinkle of almonds, and a small garnish of mint leaves.

Joyful Almond-Coconut Bars

ACTIVE TIME: **40 minutes**	INACTIVE TIME: **30 minutes**	MAKES: **24 bars**

GF

ESPRESSO ALMONDS

48 roasted salted almonds

1 tsp espresso powder

COCONUT BARS

5 cups | 400 g unsweetened finely shredded coconut

1 tsp kosher salt

1 cup | 310 g sweetened condensed milk

3 Tbsp plus 1½ tsp | 62 g coconut oil, melted

1 Tbsp plus 1½ tsp | 19 g Canna Coconut Oil (page 29), melted

CONT'D

Decorating these candy bars may be more than half the fun here. No, we take that back—eating them is still more fun, but decorating is a close second. If you want to take it up a notch, replace ¼ cup [50 g] of the chocolate chips in the coating with one Espresso Dark Chocolate Kiva Bar (60 mg CBD, 60 mg THC) from Kiva Confections, roughly chopped (see page 110).

TO MAKE THE ESPRESSO ALMONDS: Place the almonds in a small bowl and coat them lightly with butter or coconut oil baking spray. Give them a toss so the almonds have a light sheen. Add the espresso powder and toss lightly to coat. Spread the almonds in a single layer onto a plate and let dry while you prepare the coconut bars.

TO MAKE THE COCONUT BARS: Line a 9-by-13-in [23-by-33-cm] pan with parchment paper (see page 19).

In a food processor, combine the coconut and salt. Measure the sweetened condensed milk in a liquid measuring cup. Add the coconut oil and **canna coconut oil** to the cup and, using a fork or small whisk, stir until well incorporated. Pour the mixture over the shredded coconut, scraping out the sides of the cup with a rubber spatula to make sure you get it all. Process for 1 to 2 minutes until well combined, evenly coated, and the mixture resembles sticky rice.

CONT'D

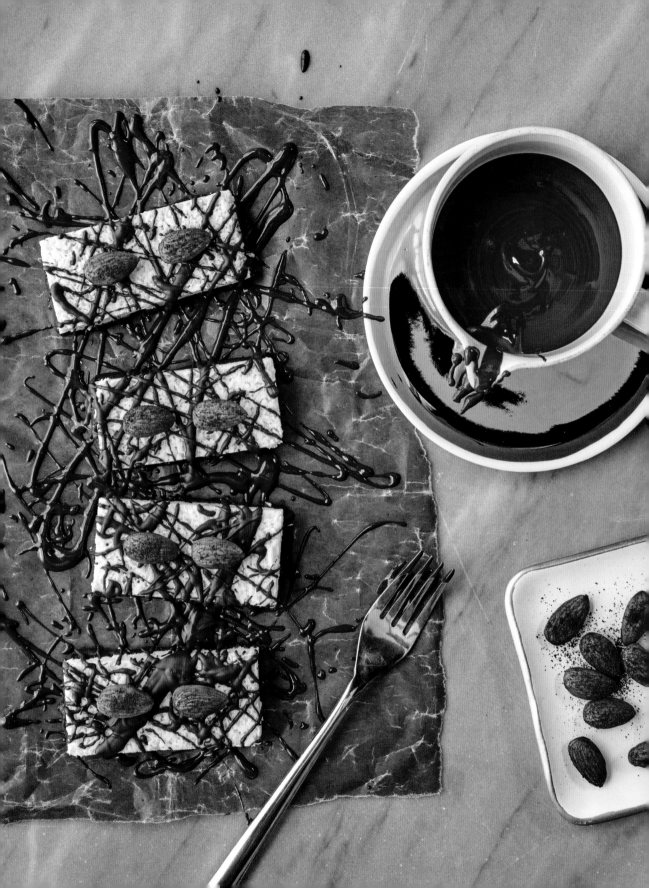

ESPRESSO CHOCOLATE COATING

2 cups | 360 g high-quality semisweet chocolate chips or féves (60% to 65% cacao)

2 tsp coconut oil, melted

2 tsp espresso powder, plus more for garnishing

SPECIAL EQUIPMENT
Double boiler (page 19)

Transfer the coconut mixture to the prepared pan and press it into an even layer using a pastry scraper or offset spatula to spread it evenly. Place a piece of parchment paper or plastic wrap on top of the mixture and use it to help press the mixture into the pan. Freeze for about 30 minutes until firm.

Line a baking sheet with parchment paper. Remove the coconut layer from the freezer and pull up on the parchment to remove it from the pan. Cut into twenty-four 1½-by-3¼-in [4-by-8-cm] bars: Divide the block into four quarters. Turn each quarter so the longer edge faces you and halve each vertically. Turn each piece so the longer edge faces you and divide each piece into thirds, vertically. Place the bars on the prepared baking sheet and return them to the freezer while you prepare the chocolate coating.

TO MAKE THE ESPRESSO CHOCOLATE COATING: In a medium heatproof bowl over a double boiler, melt together the chocolate, coconut oil, and espresso powder, stirring with a rubber spatula to combine.

Line another sheet pan with parchment paper. Remove the coconut bars from the freezer. Dip the bottom of each bar into the chocolate, shake off any excess, and place it onto the prepared sheet pan. Repeat until all bars have been dipped.

Dip the tines of a fork into the chocolate and drizzle some over the top of the bars. Let your inner Jackson Pollock go. Complete your masterpiece by topping each bar with 2 espresso-coated almonds and a final dusting of espresso powder over the entire bar. Refrigerate the bars for about 20 minutes until the chocolate hardens. Serve chilled or at room temperature. Refrigerate any leftovers in an airtight container for up to two weeks, or freeze for up to six months.

Kristi Knoblich Palmer & Scott Palmer
Kiva Confections

In 2010 Kiva Confections cofounders Scott Palmer and Kristi Knoblich Palmer started out as home kitchen entrepreneurs, running production out of the house Kristi grew up in. They put their friends and family to work, paying them in chocolate and pizza. Today, Kiva is easily one of the most recognized and respected brands in the cannabis industry, both for its socially responsible business practices, and its high-quality, trusted products.

We love Kiva chocolate bars for their consistent dosing and delicious flavors. And with their CBD bars, there's even more to love. Crafted with just the right balance of CBD to THC (1:1), these bars take chocolate therapy to a new level.

"CBD offers a great therapeutic experience," Kristi says. "Our fans asked for CBD, but we didn't want to give them just any CBD. In California, we source ours from local farms using traditional permaculture techniques. It's a safe, natural source, and we can visit the farms anytime we want."

Decadent chocolate that not only tastes good, but is good for us and ethically sourced? Yes, please. We also love how easy it is to get creative with them. From homemade medicated s'mores to candy bars like these Joyful Almond-Coconut Bars (page 107), there are countless ways to enjoy Kiva bars.

"I love shaving the espresso bar and sprinkling it over coffee," Kristi says. "The coffee aromas and the sweet chocolate come together for the perfect start to the most relaxing Saturday!"

Chocolate, cannabis, coffee . . . our happy place.

Fried Mac & Cheese Bites

| ACTIVE TIME: **1 hour, 15 minutes** | INACTIVE TIME: **3 hours** | MAKES: **16 2-by-2-in bites** |

4 oz | 115 g finely diced pancetta

2 tsp kosher salt, plus more for salting the pasta cooking water

7 oz | 200 g elbow macaroni

3¾ tsp | 16 g Canna Butter (page 27)

2 Tbsp finely diced onion

1 Tbsp minced garlic

1 cup plus 3 Tbsp | 170 g all-purpose flour

2 cups | 480 g whole milk

½ tsp freshly ground black pepper

2½ oz | 70 g crumbled gorgonzola cheese

4 oz | 115 g shredded fontina cheese

1¾ oz | 50 g shredded low-moisture mozzarella cheese

1 qt | 860 g canola oil

2 large eggs

¼ cup | 60 g water

2 cups | 120 g panko bread crumbs

I mean…fried…mac…and cheese? Mic drop. Acclaimed cannabis chef Andrea Drummer is known for creating mouthwatering dishes that are elevated on every level. These mac and cheese bites are no exception. So cheesy and gooey on the inside! So crispy and crunchy on the outside! A nod to Andrea's Southern roots, with a touch of Italian flair (hello, pancetta), this mac is comfort food at its finest. These bites take some time to prepare, but with a little planning ahead, it won't seem so bad, and it is completely worth it.

Spray an 8-by-8-in [20-by-20-cm] pan with nonstick baking spray and set aside.

In a small skillet over medium-high heat, cook the pancetta for about 5 minutes until tender and just slightly crisp. Remove 2 Tbsp of the rendered fat and set aside; if you are short, add enough vegetable, canola, or grapeseed oil to equal 2 Tbsp. Using a slotted spoon, remove the pancetta and set aside. Discard any remaining fat.

Bring a medium pot of salted water (it should taste like the sea) to a boil over high heat. Cook the macaroni for about 7 minutes until al dente. Drain and shock the pasta under cold running water.

CONT'D

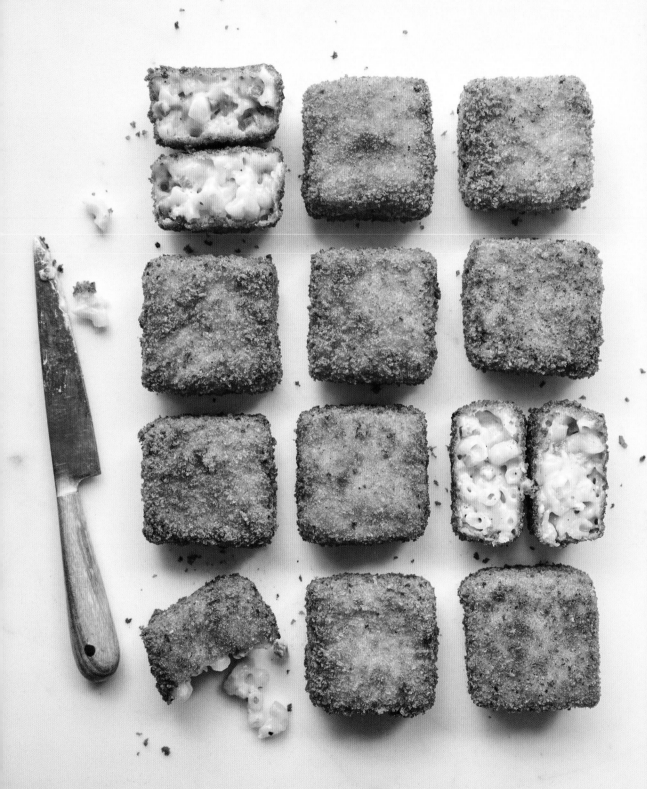

The macaroni and cheese can be made, poured into the baking dish, covered with plastic wrap, and refrigerated for up to three days before cutting, dredging, and frying.

If you're planning to serve these at a party, and want to get the frying done before guests arrive, the mac and cheese bites can be fried and left on the wire rack up to two hours at room temperature, or transferred to an airtight container and refrigerated for one day. Reheat in a 250°F [120°C] oven until warmed through and re-crisped, 20 to 30 minutes if straight from the fridge, 10 to 15 minutes if from room temperature.

Return the pot to medium heat and combine the reserved pancetta fat, **canna butter**, onion, and garlic in it. Cook, stirring, until the canna butter melts. Whisk in 3 Tbsp [30 g] of flour. Cook, whisking, for 1 to 2 minutes until the mixture is lightly browned.

While whisking to prevent lumps from forming, slowly drizzle in the milk. Add the 2 tsp salt and pepper and whisk to combine. Raise the heat to medium-high and cook for about 6 minutes until the sauce thickens and starts to bubble.

Adjust the heat to medium-low and whisk in the gorgonzola until mostly dissolved. Add the fontina, whisking until it melts and combines into the sauce. Add the mozzarella and whisk until melted and well combined. Add the pasta and pancetta to the sauce and stir well to combine.

Pour the macaroni mixture into the prepared baking pan, making sure to scrape out as much sauce as you can using a rubber spatula. Smooth the top, making sure you get the macaroni evenly into the corners of the pan. Cover with plastic wrap and refrigerate for at least 3 hours or, ideally, overnight until completely firm.

In a medium pot or deep fryer, heat the canola oil to 340°F [170°C]. Monitor the temperature with a candy thermometer clipped to the pot (if using), or drop in a few bread crumbs. If they bubble and start to brown quickly, the oil is ready. Do not let the oil get so hot that it starts smoking. Meanwhile, prepare your dredging station.

Line up 3 medium bowls: Put the remaining 1 cup [140 g] flour in the first bowl; beat together the eggs and water in the second; put the bread crumbs in the third. Line a baking sheet with parchment paper.

Remove the mac and cheese from the refrigerator. Run a paring knife around the inside edge of the pan and cut the mac into sixteen equal 2-by-2-in [5-by-5-cm] squares. Using an offset spatula or fork, remove the squares from the pan and set them aside on the prepared baking sheet.

CONT'D

Roll each macaroni square in the flour, dusting off any excess. Dredge the floured square in the egg mixture and drop it in the bread crumbs, making sure it gets a full coat of crumbs. Use one hand for flouring and the other for egging, so you don't end up breading your fingers. Place the coated square back on the baking sheet. Repeat to coat all squares.

Place a metal rack over a sheet pan and set aside. Using a large slotted metal spoon or mesh skimmer, lower a few coated pieces at a time into the hot oil. You want to work in small batches so as not to crowd the pot or drop the oil temperature too drastically. Deep-fry the bites for 1 to 2 minutes until golden brown and crispy on the outside, and hot and gooey on the inside. Transfer to a wire rack while you fry the remaining squares. Enjoy while they're still warm!

Andrea Drummer
Elevation VIP

Before Andrea Drummer became a high-end cannabis chef, she was an antidrug counselor telling high school kids to, "just say no."

"I know!" Andrea laughs. "The irony is not lost on me. After a long career in the nonprofit arena, I committed to a second career, something I have always had a passion for, culinary arts. The transition, while extreme, was the best decision I could have made." It brought her to cannabis cuisine and the creation of Elevation VIP, a Los Angeles—based company that caters intimate gourmet dinner parties.

Andrea treats cannabis like the world-class ingredient it is, masterfully pairing it with complementary flavors to create a dining experience that is, well, elevated. We love her take on the classic comfort food—mac and cheese.

"Being from the South, I grew up eating mac and cheese with different family members making it many different ways," Andrea says. "But after attending culinary school and learning classical techniques, I came to a renewed appreciation for the Southern classic. I wanted to interpret it differently by using imported cheeses outside of the familiar norm of Cheddar cheese. I've served it with étouffée, braises, and even with a unique twist on fried chicken. It has become a favorite with many clients."

We can see why. Creamy, crispy, cheesy, canna, carby. These bites are like a perfect storm of delicious satisfaction. Fried mac and cheese! You've ruined us, Andrea.

PB & J Chocolate Cups

ACTIVE TIME: **45 minutes**	INACTIVE TIME: **1 hour**	MAKES: **12 pieces**

GF

1 cup | 140 g roasted salted peanuts (see Note, page 117)

¼ cup | 78 g Canna Honey (page 34)

16 oz | 455 g high-quality semisweet chocolate chips or féves (60% to 65% cacao; about 2 cups)

2 tsp coconut oil

1 Tbsp Concord grape jelly, or your favorite jam or jelly

1 Tbsp smoked flaky sea salt (see Note, page 117)

SPECIAL EQUIPMENT
12-cup muffin pan

Double boiler (page 19)

This classic flavor combination is sure to be a crowd pleaser. A sprinkle of flaky smoked sea salt on top takes this nostalgic treat to that next level. In this recipe we show you how to make your own medicated nut butter, so have fun experimenting with different flavor combinations. Pistachio and blackberry! Almond and apricot! If you like strawberry jam (who doesn't?), use the leftover nonmedicated jam from the Strawberry Jam Pavlovas (page 126), or for a stronger dose, use medicated jam. There's no wrong way to eat these.

Line an 8-by-8-in [20-by-20-cm] pan with plastic wrap.

In a food processor, blend the peanuts for 3 to 5 minutes until smooth and creamy, pausing to scrape down the sides of the bowl a few times. Add the **canna honey**. Process until well combined, scraping down the sides once or twice more to ensure even distribution. Using a plastic spatula to scrape out every last bit, transfer the peanut butter mixture to the prepared pan. Place another sheet of plastic over the top and use your hands to spread the mixture evenly to cover the bottom of the pan. Place the pan in the freezer for 20 minutes.

CONT'D

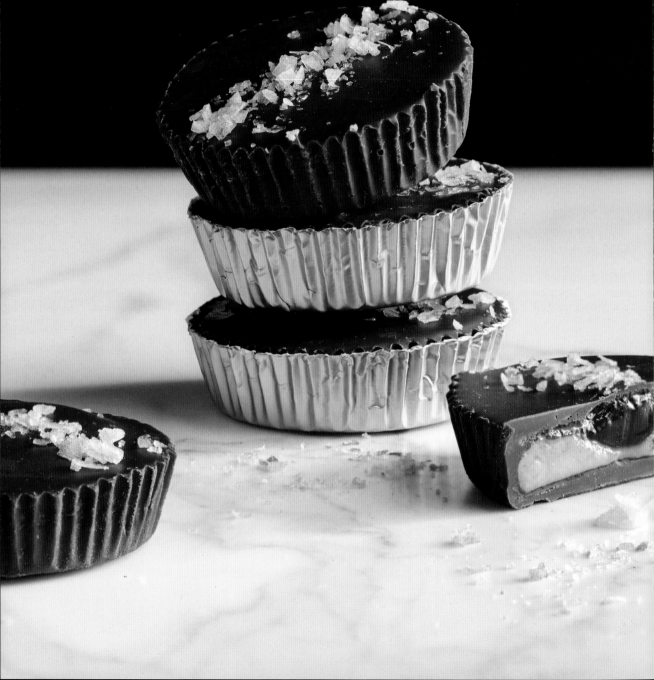

You can use store-bought natural peanut butter instead of making your own from scratch. Combine ½ cup plus 2 tsp [140 g] peanut butter and the canna honey in the bowl of a stand mixer fitted with the paddle attachment. Mix on high speed for 5 to 10 minutes, pausing to scrape down the bowl often, until thoroughly combined. Alternatively, use a handheld electric mixer to mix well.

We use Maldon sea salt whenever a recipe calls for flaky sea salt. The smoked variety used here adds a little extra something special to this treat.

Meanwhile, line a 12-cup muffin pan with cupcake liners. In a medium heatproof bowl over a double boiler, melt together the chocolate and coconut oil. Pour 1 heaping tsp of melted chocolate into the bottom of each cupcake liner. Tap and gently shake the pan a few times to make sure the bottoms of the cups are completely covered. Put the tray in the freezer so the chocolate can harden while you work with the filling. Place the remaining melted chocolate back over the double boiler to keep warm.

Remove the chilled peanut butter filling from the pan by lifting up on the plastic wrap. Cut the filling into 12 equal portions. For the most accurate dosage, weigh the total amount of peanut butter filling and divide by twelve to determine the target weight of filling per serving (about 18 g). Roll each portion into a ball and flatten it into a disc about 1½ in [4 cm] in diameter.

Remove the muffin tray from the freezer. Place 1 peanut butter disc into the center of each cup. You should have a scant ⅛-in [4-mm] gap between the edge of the peanut butter and the edge of the chocolate bottom. This gap ensures the peanut butter is completely enclosed once you add chocolate on top. Make an indent in the center of the peanut butter using the back of a ¼-tsp measure. Spoon ¼ tsp of grape jelly into each indent.

Equally divide the remaining melted chocolate among the muffin cups, about 2 tsp per cup. Once covered, tap the muffin tray onto the counter a few times to make sure the chocolate settles down the sides of the cups. Use a toothpick or a small knife to push the chocolate down the sides, if necessary.

Refrigerate for 10 minutes. Remove and sprinkle the top of each peanut butter cup with ¼ tsp of smoked sea salt. Refrigerate again for about 1 hour until the chocolate is completely set. Keep the cups refrigerated in an airtight container for up to one month, or in the freezer for up to six months.

Mexican Street Corn & Cheese Crisps

ACTIVE TIME: **1 hour, 45 minutes**	INACTIVE TIME: **10 minutes**	MAKES: **24 corn cups**

GF

CRISPY PARMESAN CUPS
One 20-oz | 570-g package grated (not shredded) Parmigiano-Reggiano cheese

CORN FILLING
2 ears fresh sweet corn, husks and silks removed, each ear wrapped individually in aluminum foil

1 small shallot, finely diced

¼ cup | 35 g packed crumbled Cotija cheese

¼ cup | 10 g finely chopped fresh cilantro

1 Tbsp freshly squeezed lime juice

½ tsp kosher salt

¼ tsp freshly ground black pepper

CONT'D

Cannabis chef Monica Lo has a way of creating canna-infused recipes that get you so inspired and excited you just want to run into the kitchen and try all the things. When we first came across her fresh cannabis chimichurri recipe (which uses raw nonpsychoactive cannabis leaves as a flavor component), our wheels started turning. We love this medicated chimichurri in our fancy-pants take on *elotes,* a classic Mexican street food of grilled corn slathered in cheese, chile, and lime. All the punchy flavors are there, but we take the corn off the cob, and into crispy irresistible Parmesan cups.

TO MAKE THE CRISPY PARMESAN CUPS: Preheat the oven to 375°F [190°C]. Line two sheet pans with parchment paper or silicone baking mats and spray them with nonstick baking spray.

On one prepared sheet pan, place 2 Tbsp [10 g] of Parmigiano-Reggiano cheese and gently smooth the mound into a flat circle approximately 4 in [10 cm] in diameter. Place 1 Tbsp [5 g] of Parmigiano-Reggiano cheese in the center of the circle, leaving it in a mound. Repeat until you have six circles on the prepared sheet. Bake for 8 to 10 minutes until the cheese is golden brown and pliable.

As one batch bakes, get the next batch ready to bake on the second prepared sheet.

CONT'D

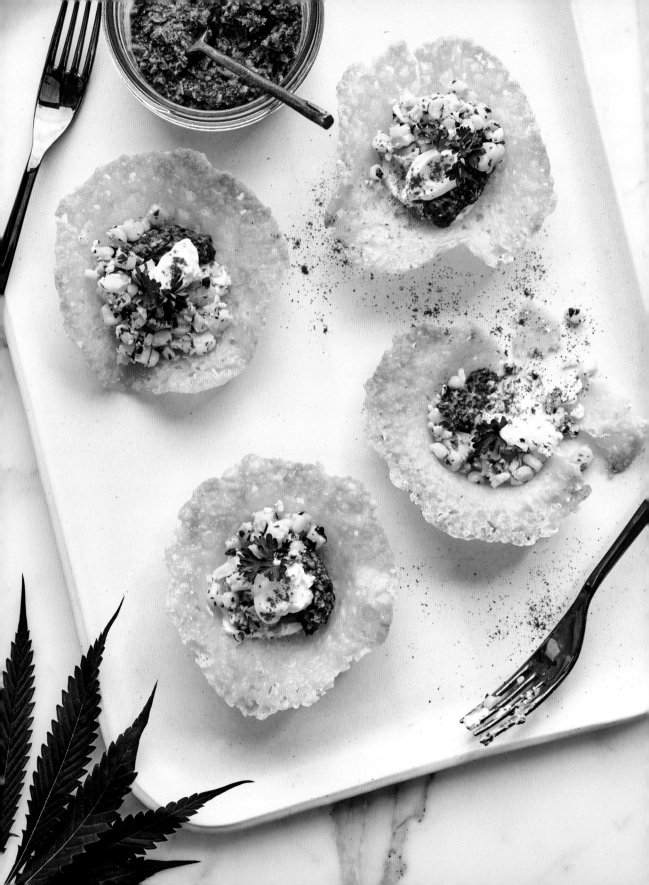

CHIMICHURRI SPREAD

1 garlic clove

1 small | 30 g shallot

¼ cup | 10 g finely chopped flat-leaf parsley

½ small | 6 g red jalapeño, seeded

3 Tbsp | 9 g finely chopped raw cannabis leaves, stems removed, or fresh cilantro

3 Tbsp | 9 g finely chopped fresh cilantro

2 Tbsp red wine vinegar

2 Tbsp | 20 g pepitas

1 Tbsp plus 1½ tsp | 19 g Canna Coconut Oil (page 29), melted

1 Tbsp plus 1½ tsp extra-virgin olive oil

1½ tsp freshly squeezed lime juice

¼ tsp kosher salt

FINISHING TOUCHES

Sour cream for garnishing

Chili powder for garnishing

SPECIAL EQUIPMENT

12-cup muffin pan

When batch one is done, working quickly, use a small spatula to transfer the cheese circles onto an inverted muffin tin. Gently mold the circles to the shape of the muffin cups. If the cheese is too hot to handle, use a paper towel to protect your fingers. The cups will start to harden quickly. Let the Parmesan cups cool until firm and crisp.

Repeat with the next batch, and continue until you have twenty-four cups.

TO MAKE THE CORN FILLING: Preheat the grill to medium-high heat or the oven to 375°F [190°C].

Grill the foil-wrapped corn for 15 to 20 minutes, rotating frequently. The corn should be lightly charred and cooked all the way through. Alternatively, roast the corn in the oven for about 25 minutes. Let sit until cool enough to handle.

Using a serrated knife, cut the corn kernels off the cobs into a large bowl. Add the shallot, Cotija, cilantro, lime juice, salt, and pepper. Stir to combine. Set aside until assembly time.

TO MAKE THE CHIMICHURRI SPREAD: In a food processor, combine all the chimichurri ingredients and process until smooth. Scrape down the sides of the bowl with a rubber spatula as needed to process the ingredients evenly.

TO ASSEMBLE: Take a crispy Parmigiano-Reggiano cup and spread a bit of sour cream on the bottom of the cup. Spread 1 tsp [5 g] chimichurri on top of the sour cream. Evenly divide the corn filling among the cups (each cup should get about 1½ Tbsp). Top each cup with a small dollop of sour cream and a dash of chili powder. Enjoy immediately.

Monica Lo
Sous Weed

Monica Lo is the chef-founder of Sous Weed, where she has carved out a unique intersection of cannabis, food, and creative content. As fellow food nerds, we fell in love with Monica's approach to cooking with cannabis, and her use of sous vide techniques has both inspired and guided us in our own sous weed experiments (see Sous Vide Canna Infusions, page 31).

Monica knows a thing or two about sous vide cooking. Before cannabis was her full-time job, she was the creative director and ran the test kitchen at Nomiku, a startup that builds hardware and software for easy sous vide cooking. "Since you're cooking underwater at a very precise temperature, sous vide lends itself perfectly to cannabis cooking,"

Monica explains. "It's consistent, it's discreet, and it's so simple—just set it and forget it!"

Beyond basic infusions, Monica's recipes are creative, modern, and delicious. "Cannabis is a tasty, versatile, nutrient-dense plant, and we should treat it as a culinary challenge like any other," she says. "I really believe in the use of cannabis as an ingredient, as opposed to merely a psychoactive additive. In fact, I love using fresh cannabis leaves. Raw cannabis can give you a ton of health benefits without the psychoactive components you'd normally experience when heating the plant. I've even played around with juicing it."

Cannabis—the new kale! Imagine that.

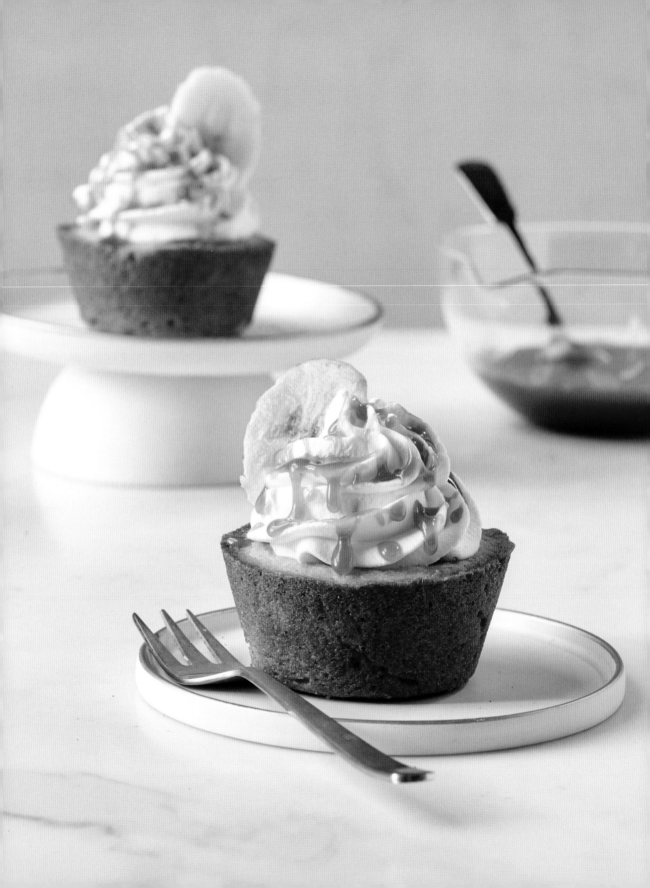

Banana Cream & Salted Caramel Cookie Cups

ACTIVE TIME: **1 hour, 30 minutes** | INACTIVE TIME: **10 minutes** | MAKES: **12 cookie cups**

Banana cream pie gets a novel makeover with a cookie cup crust and a decadent drizzle of salted caramel. Once you've mastered the technique of making these cookie cups, you may be tempted to turn every cookie recipe into its own little edible vessel. The salted caramel and banana cream combination is a winner, but chocolate and banana is no slouch either! If you're so inclined, for a stronger dose, substitute a spoonful of Chocolate Hazelnut Spread (page 42) for the salted caramel.

VANILLA COOKIE CUPS

5 oz | 140 g unsalted butter, at room temperature

2 tsp | 9 g Canna Butter, at room temperature (page 27)

²/₃ cup | 130 g sugar

1 Tbsp vanilla extract

1 Tbsp honey

½ tsp kosher salt

¼ tsp baking soda

4 large egg yolks

2 cups plus 2½ Tbsp | 305 g all-purpose flour

¹/₃ cup | 80 g heavy cream

PASTRY CREAM

1 cup | 240 g whole milk

3 Tbsp plus 1½ tsp | 45 g sugar

¼ tsp kosher salt

CONT'D

TO MAKE THE VANILLA COOKIE: Preheat the oven to 325°F (165°C).

In a bowl of a stand mixer fitted with the paddle attachment, or in a large bowl with a handheld mixer, combine the butter, **canna butter**, sugar, vanilla, honey, salt, and baking soda. Cream the mixture for about 5 minutes on medium speed until light and fluffy, pausing about halfway through the mixing to scrape down the sides of the bowl with a rubber spatula. With the mixer still running add the egg yolks, one at a time, mixing until one is incorporated before adding the next. Scrape down the sides of the bowl again. Turn the mixer to low speed and add the flour all at once. Slowly bring the speed up to medium as the flour is incorporated. With the mixer running, drizzle in the cream. Mix until combined, scraping down the sides once more to make sure all ingredients are evenly incorporated. Pop the bowl into the refrigerator for 10 minutes so the dough can firm up a little.

CONT'D

1 Tbsp plus 1½ tsp cornstarch

1 large egg

1 large egg yolk

1 Tbsp unsalted butter

½ tsp vanilla bean paste
or vanilla extract

FINISHING TOUCHES

1 cup | 240 g heavy cream

2 medium bananas, ripe but
still firm

¼ cup | 82 g caramel sauce

Kosher salt

SPECIAL EQUIPMENT

12-cup muffin pan

Shot glass

Pastry bag (optional)

Coat a 12-cup muffin pan with nonstick baking spray. Form the dough into 12 equal balls (see Note). For the most accurate dosage, weigh the total amount of dough and divide by twelve to determine the target weight per serving (about 51 g). Coat your hands with cooking spray to keep the dough from sticking to them as you form the balls. Place the balls into the muffin pan and press down to flatten the dough into the cups just so they cover the bottoms.

Place the muffin pan on a baking sheet. Bake for 17 to 20 minutes until the cookies are lightly browned and mostly set. Rotate the pan halfway through the baking time to ensure even cooking.

TO MAKE THE PASTRY CREAM: While the cookies bake, in a medium saucepan over medium heat, combine the milk, 2 Tbsp of sugar, and the salt. Cook for about 4 minutes until steamy and a few small bubbles start to rise to the surface.

In a small bowl, whisk the remaining 1 Tbsp plus 1½ tsp sugar and the cornstarch. In a medium bowl, whisk the whole egg and egg yolk. Add the cornstarch mixture to the eggs and whisk until well combined. When the milk is ready, remove it from the heat and slowly pour it into the egg mixture, whisking constantly. Transfer this mixture back to the saucepan and simmer for 2 to 5 minutes over medium-low heat, whisking constantly, until it reaches the consistency of thick pudding.

Remove the saucepan from the heat and stir in the butter and vanilla. If the mixture isn't quite as smooth as you'd like, run it through a fine-mesh sieve. Pour the pastry cream into a shallow bowl. Place plastic wrap directly on the surface to prevent a skin from forming, and refrigerate it for about 30 minutes to chill completely.

NOTE

Using a scale to portion the dough is highly recommended for this recipe, however, if you do not have a scale, portion the dough using a ¼-cup [60-ml] dry measure or 2-oz [55-g] scoop. Level the scoop when measuring, and scrape out all of the dough from the scoop each time.

MAKE-AHEAD TIP

The pastry cream can be made up to three days in advance, but wait to add the mashed banana until right before assembling. Make sure it is covered with plastic wrap touching the surface so a skin doesn't form.

TO FORM THE COOKIE CUPS: Spray the outside of a shot glass with baking spray. Remove the cookies when the time is up, and leave the oven on. Using the shot glass, carefully press down into the center of each cookie and gently spin the glass to create a well. In a circular motion, press the shot glass against the sides of the cup to widen the well. Try to create as deep a well as possible without breaking the cookie—be deliberate, yet cautious. Once the cups are formed, return the pan to the oven for 6 to 8 minutes more until the centers are set and the cookies are golden.

Remove the pan from the oven and let the cookie cups sit in the pan for 10 minutes. Run a paring knife around the edge of the cookie cups to loosen them and invert the pan over a wire cooling rack, letting the cookie cups fall out. Cool completely.

TO ASSEMBLE: In a large bowl, whip the cream to medium peaks by hand with a whisk or with the help of a handheld electric mixer. Set aside.

Take the pastry cream out of the fridge. Mash one-half to three-fourths of a banana with a fork into a purée. Stir it into the pastry cream until evenly incorporated. Transfer the banana pastry cream to a pastry bag or resealable plastic bag with a corner snipped off to about a ¾-in [2-cm] opening. (This step is optional, but we find it is the easiest and cleanest way to fill the cups.)

Warm the caramel sauce to a pourable consistency in a microwave-safe container in the microwave for 30 seconds on high power, or in a small saucepan over medium heat for about 3 minutes on the stovetop. Season it to taste with salt.

Cut the remaining banana into ¼-in [6-mm] slices. Place one slice into the bottom of each cookie cup. Drizzle in about 1 tsp caramel. Fill each cup to the brim with about 1 Tbsp [15 g] pastry cream. Top with whipped cream and a final drizzle of caramel. Garnish with another banana slice. Enjoy immediately.

Strawberry Jam Pavlovas

| ACTIVE TIME: **2 hours** | INACTIVE TIME: **4 hours** | MAKES: **24 Pavlovas** |

GF

AQUAFABA VANILLA MERINGUES

1 Tbsp cornstarch

1 Tbsp freshly squeezed lemon juice

1 tsp vanilla extract

²/₃ cup | 150 g aquafaba (canned chickpea liquid), from one or two chilled 15-oz | 430-g cans chickpeas

1 cup plus 2 Tbsp | 230 g sugar

CONT'D

These mini Pavlovas are lovely, unexpected, and just a little edgy. Ethereal, light, vanilla meringues made with aquafaba (chickpea water!) come together like magic (and without the slightest hint of beaniness). For the jam in these Pavlovas, we went straight to the experts. Our friends at Flour Child make some of the best jam around, and this homemade strawberry number spiked with a touch of black pepper is the star of the show. A dollop of tangy whipped cream and a drizzle of balsamic reduction tie it all together to make one unforgettable dessert.

TO MAKE THE AQUAFABA VANILLA MERINGUES: Preheat the oven to 200°F [95°C]. Line two baking sheets with parchment paper or silicone baking mats.

In a small bowl, mix together the cornstarch, lemon juice, and vanilla. Set aside.

Remove the chickpeas from the fridge and strain them, reserving the liquid (a.k.a. aquafaba). Reserve the beans for another use (like vibrant Roasted Beet Hummus, page 45). Place ²/₃ cup [150 g] of the liquid in the bowl of a stand mixer fitted with the whisk attachment. Beat the aquafaba for 1 to 2 minutes on medium-high speed until the liquid becomes thickened and foamy.

CONT'D

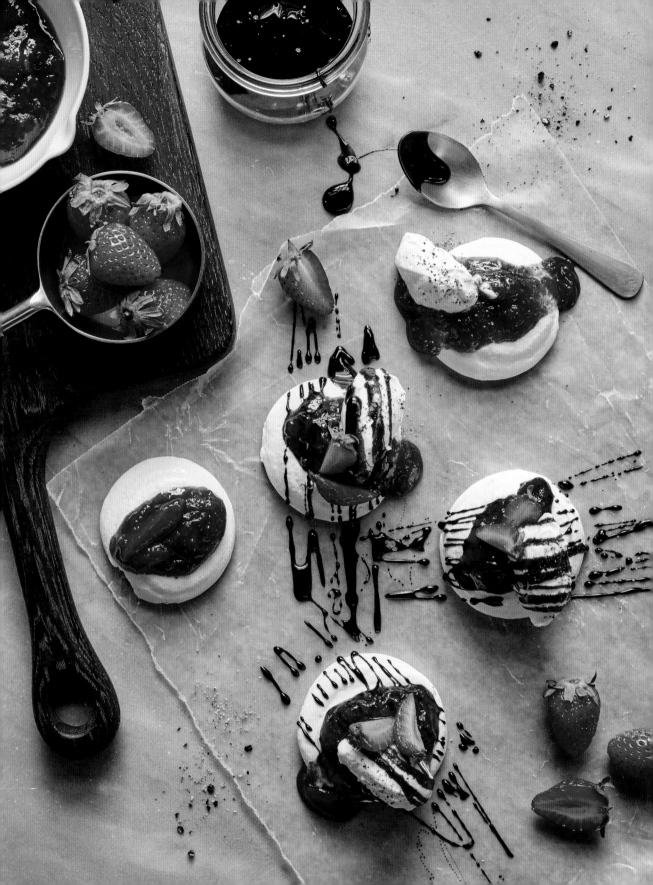

STRAWBERRY BLACK PEPPER JAM (SEE NOTE)

2 pt | 350 g fresh strawberries, hulled and quartered

¼ cup plus 2 Tbsp | 80 g organic cane sugar

Peel of ½ lemon

½ split vanilla bean, seeds scraped

¼ tsp freshly ground black pepper, plus more for garnishing

2 Tbsp honey

1 Tbsp plus 1½ tsp | 20 g Canna Coconut Oil (page 29)

BALSAMIC GLAZE

1 cup | 265 g balsamic vinegar

2 Tbsp packed brown sugar

YOGURT CREAM

1 cup | 240 g heavy cream

1 cup | 240 g plain full-fat Greek yogurt

2 Tbsp honey

SPECIAL EQUIPMENT

Pastry bag and round tip

With the mixer running, gradually add the sugar in 2 to 3 increments. Once all the sugar is added, crank up the speed to high and beat for about 9 minutes until the mixture triples in volume and holds stiff peaks. Turn the speed to low and add the cornstarch mixture. Return the speed to high for about 30 seconds until you have an airy, glossy meringue that holds a stiff peak when you remove the whisk attachment.

Transfer the meringue to a pastry bag with a round tip (Ateco 805) or resealable plastic bag with a corner snipped off to form a ½-in [12-mm] opening. Pipe tight 2-in [5-cm] coils onto the prepared sheets. Continue piping on top of each circle, just around the outer edge, to create a little wall surrounding it. Leave about 3 in [7.5 cm] between each meringue so they have room to spread as they bake.

Bake the meringues for 2½ to 3½ hours until they are completely dry, hard to the touch, and peel easily off the baking sheets. Transfer to a wire cooling rack to cool completely. Transfer the meringues to an airtight container as soon as they are cooled so they stay dry and crisp. (If you leave them out too long and they become sticky, return them to a 200°F [95°C] oven until they dry out again.) Meanwhile, prepare the other components.

TO MAKE THE STRAWBERRY BLACK PEPPER JAM: Place a small plate in the freezer. In a medium saucepan, combine the strawberries and sugar.

Using a sharp paring knife, scrape away as much of the white pith as possible from the lemon peel. Cut the peel crosswise into small, thin pieces. Add the pieces of lemon peel to the berries in the pan, along with the vanilla bean, pepper, and honey. Mix well, squishing the berries with your hands and distributing everything evenly.

Place the pan over medium-high heat, stirring occasionally, until the mixture comes to a boil, 8 to 10 minutes. Adjust the heat to medium-low and cook the mixture for 20 to 30 minutes until it is thickened, jammy, and reduced by about half (a little less than 1 cup [about 300 g]). Stir occasionally, scraping down the sides of the pan with a rubber spatula. Don't skim off the foam.

When your jam looks ready, remove the plate from the freezer and drop a spoonful of hot jam on it to check for doneness. Let it cool for 1 to 2 minutes to test the texture. If the jam is done, it will gel up. If it is too runny, continue cooking for a few minutes more and test again.

To save some time, dress up store-bought jam instead of making it from scratch: In a small saucepan over low heat, warm ½ cup [150 g] of strawberry jam until it is a pourable consistency. Remove the pan from the heat and add the canna coconut oil and a pinch of black pepper. Whisk vigorously until thoroughly combined. Or, use Flour Child's (see page 130) medicated jam for a stronger dose.

MAKE-AHEAD TIP

The aquafaba meringues can be made ahead and stored in an airtight container at room temperature for up to two weeks, longer if you include food-grade desiccant packets in the container. The strawberry black pepper jam can be made ahead and refrigerated in an airtight container for up to two weeks, and much longer if you properly can it. The balsamic glaze can be made ahead and stored in an airtight container at room temperature for up to one day. The yogurt cream can be made and refrigerated in an airtight container for up to one day.

VARIATION

Have fun with the flavor profile of the strawberry jam! Not into black pepper? Play with fresh herbs, like verbena or tarragon. Rose geranium is lovely; a splash of orange-flavored liqueur such as Grand Marnier is divine.

Remove and discard the vanilla bean (remember to squeeze out all the goodness first!). Measure ½ cup [150 g] of jam into a liquid measuring cup. Add the **canna coconut oil** and stir vigorously until melted and well combined. Transfer this medicated jam to an airtight container and clearly label it. Keep refrigerated until the Pavlovas are ready to assemble. Reserve the remaining jam for other uses (stir it into seltzer with a splash of cream to make a homemade Italian soda, or use it in the fun PB & J Chocolate Cups, page 115). It can be infused or left unmedicated—dealer's choice. Transfer it to an airtight container, label it, and refrigerate for up to two weeks.

TO MAKE THE BALSAMIC GLAZE: In a small saucepan over medium-high heat, combine the balsamic vinegar and brown sugar. Bring to a boil, adjust the heat to low, and simmer for about 15 minutes, stirring occasionally, until the liquid is reduced to a syrupy consistency thick enough to coat the back of a spoon.

TO MAKE THE YOGURT CREAM: In the bowl of a stand mixer fitted with the whisk attachment, or in a large bowl with a handheld mixer, combine the cream, yogurt, and honey. Beat for 3 to 5 minutes on medium-high speed until the mixture holds stiff peaks.

TO ASSEMBLE: Take a meringue and fill the well with 1 tsp [6 g] of strawberry black pepper jam. Top with a dollop of whipped yogurt cream and a drizzle of balsamic glaze. Finish with a crack of black pepper. Enjoy!

Stephany Gocobachi & Akhil Khadse
Flour Child

Born and raised in San Francisco, Stephany was seduced by the magic of food from a young age. She took over Thanksgiving dinner at the ripe age of eight. Then came the equally magical discovery of cannabis at fifteen—and nothing has been the same since. Stephany enlisted her culinary prowess and created medicated delights like "mac and trees" and homemade black-and-white cookies to sell at school. Even then, she asked herself, "Why do people only make brownies?"

On her eighteenth birthday, Stephany promptly acquired a medical card and giddily walked into her first dispensary. Sadly, she was extremely disappointed by everything—from packaging to taste to the quality of cannabis used. "There was such a disconnect with the food culture of San Francisco," says Stephany. "A lot of what was on the market was not real food. They were made with ingredients that weren't fresh. I bought so many edibles that were not edible, time and time again. That was when I knew this is what I wanted to do for

a living—and I wanted to learn how to do it at the highest level I could."

Fast-forward to today: We'd say she is doing just that. Together with her partner, Akhil Khadse, Stephany created Flour Child, and has been raising the bar for cannabis edibles ever since. Their signature seasonal jam and granola are made with organic ingredients and strain-specific, whole-flower rosin pressed in house. The jams are made in small batches, with real, whole, fresh fruit harvested at its peak from local farms. "I believe that things should be enjoyed at their peak. Otherwise, what's the point?"

We could not agree more, Stephany. And trust us, we have been enjoying the heck out of your strawberry jam. We love how versatile it is. When we're not making gorgeous Pavlovas with it, we love to stir it into Coconut Yogurt (page 69) or spread it in fancy grilled cheese. Peak enjoyment, indeed.

Blueberry Lemon Macarons

ACTIVE TIME: **1 hour** | INACTIVE TIME: **1 hour, 20 minutes** | MAKES: **25 macarons**

GF

LEMON CURD

1 Tbsp packed lemon zest, from 2 to 3 Meyer lemons or regular lemons

½ cup | 120 ml freshly squeezed lemon juice, from 2 to 3 Meyer lemons or regular lemons

3 large eggs

¼ cup plus 2 Tbsp | 80 g sugar

¼ tsp kosher salt

5 Tbsp | 75 g unsalted butter, cut into ½-in [12-mm] pieces

1 Tbsp + 1 tsp | 17g Canna Butter (page 27)

CONT'D

These exquisite French macarons are the ultimate highbrow edible. Filled with a bright, creamy lemon curd and surprise blueberry inclusion, these macarons are the loveliest. They may take a little practice to master, but, once you do, and you whip up a batch of these for your friends? Boom. That's the sound of some minds being blown.

TO MAKE THE LEMON CURD: Fill a medium saucepan with 1 to 2 in [3 to 5 cm] of water and bring it barely to a simmer over medium-high heat. Adjust the heat to low.

In a medium heatproof bowl, combine the lemon zest and juice. Add the eggs, sugar, and salt. Whisk for about 1 minute until pale yellow and a bit frothy. Set the bowl over the saucepan (the bottom of the bowl shouldn't touch the surface of the water). Add the unsalted butter, a few pieces at a time, whisking until the butter melts. Whisk in the **canna butter**. Continue to cook for about 10 minutes, whisking frequently, until the mixture thickens and you see a few bubbles come to the surface. The lemon curd should be thick enough that when you lift your whisk and let the curd drizzle into the bowl, it leaves a trail on the surface.

CONT'D

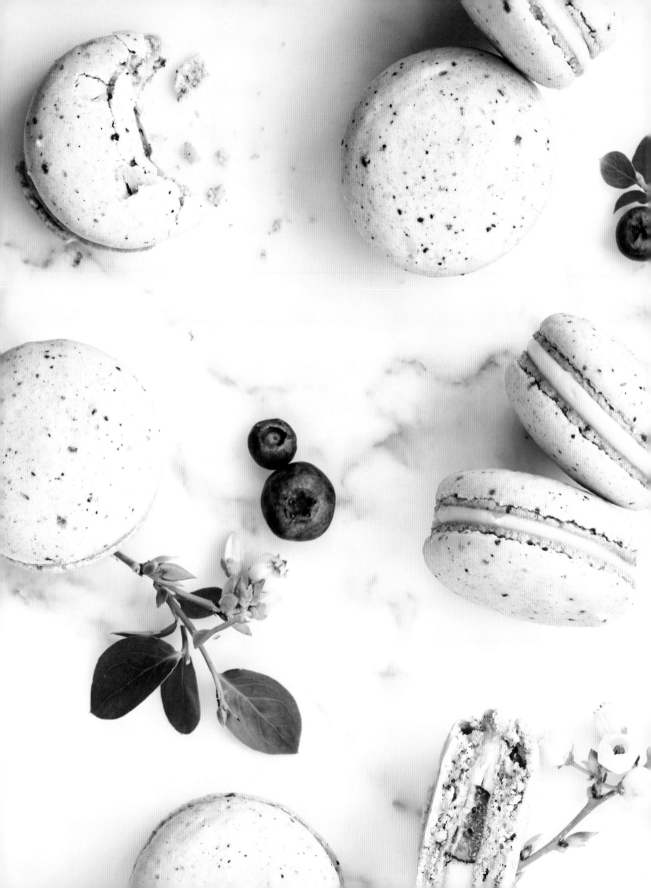

BLUEBERRY MACARON SHELLS

¼ cup plus 1 Tbsp | 9 g freeze-dried blueberries

1 ²/₃ cups | 200 g powdered sugar

1 cup | 120 g almond meal

¼ tsp kosher salt

½ cup | 100 g sugar

¹/₈ tsp cream of tartar

5¼ oz | 150 g egg whites, from 4 to 5 large eggs, at room temperature

25 fresh blueberries

SPECIAL EQUIPMENT

2 macaron piping guides (page 20)

Pastry bag and decorative tip (page 20)

Set a fine-mesh sieve over a medium bowl. Remove the lemon curd from the heat and wipe the bottom of the bowl with a clean towel. Pour the curd into the sieve, using a rubber spatula to scrape out the bowl. Strain the curd, using the rubber spatula to stir and help pass it through. Place plastic wrap directly on the surface to prevent a skin from forming, and refrigerate for at least two hours to chill completely.

TO MAKE THE BLUEBERRY MACARON SHELLS: Preheat the oven to 290°F [145°C]. Line two baking sheets with parchment paper or silicone baking mats. To help you pipe same-size circles, use guides, placed beneath your parchment paper or baking mats (you'll be able to see the circles through the parchment when it's time to pipe).

In a food processor, process the freeze-dried blueberries to a powder. Add the powdered sugar, almond meal, and salt. Process just until everything is well combined, pausing to scrape down the bowl a few times. Set aside.

In a small bowl, whisk the sugar and cream of tartar together.

Place the egg whites in the bowl of a stand mixer fitted with the whisk attachment. Beat for 1 to 2 minutes on medium-high speed until soft peaks form. Turn the speed to low, and slowly add the sugar and cream of tartar mixture. Bring the speed back up to medium-high and continue to beat for 3 to 5 minutes until the mixture holds medium peaks. To test the peaks: Stop the mixer, remove the whisk attachment, dip it into the whites, and lift it out. The peak should hold its shape, with the tip curling over on itself.

CONT'D

MAKE-AHEAD TIP

The lemon curd can be made ahead and stored in an airtight container for up to one week. Filled macarons can be refrigerated in an airtight container for up to one week, or in the freezer for up to three months. Thaw at room temperature for about 5 minutes before enjoying.

Remove the bowl from the stand mixer. Place a fine-mesh sieve over the bowl and sift in half of the almond meal mixture from the food processor. Using a rubber spatula, fold the ingredients until just combined. Sift in the remaining almond meal mixture. Continue folding, 60 to 70 folds, until the mixture is evenly combined and has the consistency of a gooey cake batter. To test for doneness, lift the spatula and drizzle a ribbon of batter into the bowl. The macaron batter should have enough body to hold its shape, but enough fluidity that the ribbon relaxes into the batter after sitting for a minute. If it is too stiff and doesn't have that "melting" quality, the batter needs more folding.

Transfer the macaron batter to a pastry bag fitted with a plain tip (Ateco 804 or Wilton 2A) or a resealable plastic bag with $1/3$ in [8 mm] snipped off a bottom corner.

Take your prepared baking sheets and dab a bit of batter to the underside of the parchment so it stays put. On each tray, pipe twenty-five 1½-in [4-cm] circles using the stencil guides: Hold the tip of the pastry bag at an angle to the baking sheet and squeeze to pipe your circles. As you reach the desired size, stop squeezing, and make a quick flicking motion like the shape of a comma as you lift up the tip. Remove the circle guideline before baking.

Place a dishtowel on the counter. Grabbing both sides of the pan, lightly tap the pan on the towel a few times to dislodge any air bubbles lurking beneath the surface, waiting for the opportunity to crack your precious macarons. If any bubbles rise that don't pop on their own, use a toothpick to help them along. Do this immediately after piping to allow the holes to smooth out while they dry. Let the macaron shells rest for 20 to 30 minutes, or until dry to the touch, ideally with an oscillating fan in the room. Macarons are infamous for being fickle, depending on weather and humidity. Don't make macarons on a rainy day.

Bake one tray at a time for 18 to 20 minutes, rotating the tray halfway through the baking time. Do not let the macaron shells brown. To check for doneness, lift a corner of the parchment paper and carefully slide a finger underneath the paper and a macaron while gently peeling the paper back. The bottom should be flat and peel off easily. The top should not give when lightly tapped with your fingertip. Do not check for doneness more than once or twice during baking—opening and closing the oven causes the temperature to drop, which could cause the cookies to collapse. When the cookies are done, transfer them, on the parchment paper, to cooling racks, and cool completely before peeling off the paper.

TO ASSEMBLE: Pair macaron shells of similar size. Remove the lemon curd from the refrigerator and transfer it to a pastry bag or resealable plastic bag with a bottom corner snipped off to form a ½-in [12-mm] opening. For the most accurate dosage, weigh the total amount of lemon curd and divide it by twenty-five to determine the target weight per serving (about 15 g). Place a macaron half (bottom-side up) on the scale, tare the weight, and then pipe until you reach the target weight. Alternately, squeeze the filling to the size of a quarter (about 1 Tbsp) onto the center of the shell (bottom-side up). Repeat until you've piped 25 halves.

Place a blueberry in the center of the lemon curd on each cookie half and gently press the matching macaron mate (bottom-side down) on top of the filling to make a little sandwich. Be careful not to let the filling ooze out the edges. Transfer the assembled macarons to an airtight container and refrigerate at least two hours before serving. Impress the pants off someone by offering them the fanciest edible they've ever seen.

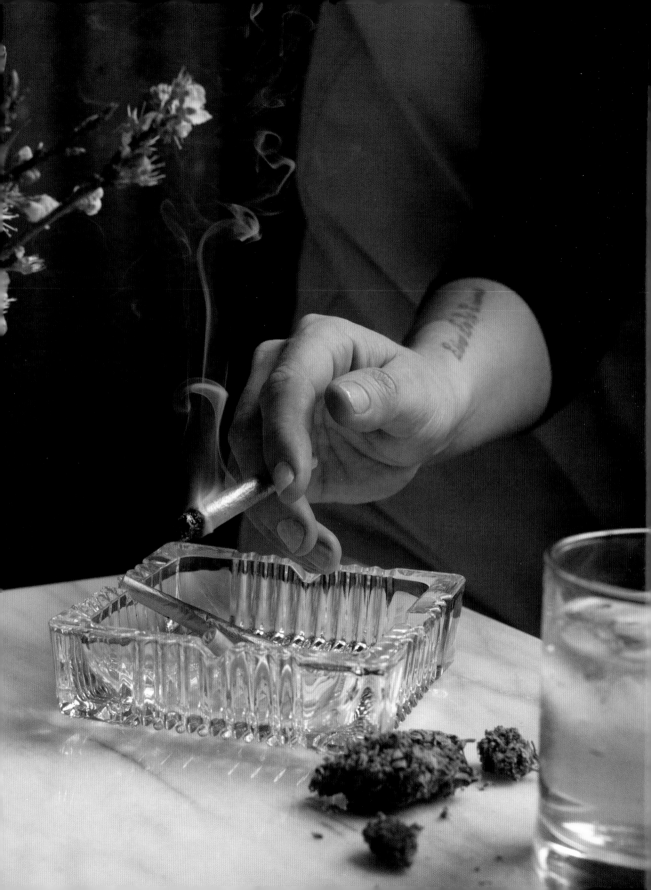

Outro

Acknowledgments

First, immense gratitude to cannabis. You brought us here and have become an inextricable part of our lives. Thank you for being magical.

Special thanks to Hua and Ryan. For running all the errands, and tasting all the things, and keeping our spirits high, and for believing in us, always. This book would not be possible without you. We love you.

Huge thank yous to our amazing recipe testers: Sheri Codiana and Emily McFarren, you guys are recipe-testing machines. Thank you for your tireless work, your thoughtful feedback, and your never-ending enthusiasm. Thank you to Margie Kriebel, Patty Ponciano, Lisa Rossi, and Scott Weiss for lending us your very capable hands. You guys saved us.

Special thanks to Andrea Burnett and The 4Twenty Group, LLC, our champion and consigliere. We are so grateful to you for bringing this incredible opportunity to us. Your support throughout this process has been invaluable.

Thank you to Jodi Liano for being the consummate connector you are, for introducing us to Andrea in the first place, and for making your dream come true so we could make ours come true.

Thank you to San Francisco Cooking School for playing such an integral role in how we got here. Thank you, Catherine Pantsios, for preparing us. Thank you, Nicole Plue, for your guidance and incredible knowledge.

Thank you to Aaron Flynn and Neil Dellacava at Gold Seal for coming through on getting us the best ingredients. We really enjoyed it.

Thank you to Tyson Graham for your dedication to your craft. Your work powered much of this book.

Thank you to all the gifted makers who contributed to this book: Andrea Drummer, Kenny Morrison, Leone Posod and Cindy Pinzon, Maya Elisabeth and Whoopi Goldberg, Monica Lo, Scott Palmer and Kristi Knoblich Palmer, Stephany Gocobachi and Akhil Khadse, you inspire us and we have so much hope for the future of our industry knowing such passionate, creative, and talented people are driving it.

Thank you to Emily Richardson and the CW Analytical team for your support and expertise. We know we can always count on you.

Thank you to Sarah Malarkey at Chronicle for believing in us, and to Lizzie Vaughan and Sahara Clement for all your hard work. To Mary Cassells for your thoughtful reading and editing, this is a better book thanks to you. Thank you to Linda Xiao, Glenn Jenkins, Sherese Elsey, and Zach Wine for making us look good.

Thank you to the Meadow family for cheering us on and for being such enthusiastic guinea pigs.

Mom and Dad, thank you for your unconditional love and support. You've given me every opportunity and raised me to believe I can accomplish anything. You are my heroes.

And Hazel, thank you, baby girl, for taking good naps and sleeping through the night so Mama could write a cookbook.

Resources

CW ANALYTICAL
All potency testing for this book was done with our partners at CW Analytical, an independent quality assurance laboratory. CW Analytical provides patients, cultivators, producers, and dispensaries with important information about the safety, quality, and potency of their medical cannabis products. *cwanalytical.com*

GOLD SEAL
Gold Seal provided us with premium indoor cannabis flower for our recipe testing. Their quality products and exotic strains can be found in various dispensaries in California. *goldsealsf.com*

MEADOW
Meadow is a full-service technology company for the cannabis industry. As a consumer, Meadow allows you to browse menus of dispensaries located near you and order quality cannabis delivered right to your door in 1 hour or less. They also have a program that allows you to consult with a licensed physician and obtain a medical cannabis card via video chat. *getmeadow.com*

NOMIKU
Nomiku is a home sous vide machine that allows you to precisely control the time and temperature of what you're cooking—cannabis or otherwise. It is particularly useful in creating cannabis infusions because of its level of precision, hands-off method, and discretion. *nomiku.com*

NOVA BY ARDENT
The NOVA is a precise, and discrete, decarb device for people who want to make their own edibles at home. You simply place your raw flower in the device, seal the lid, hit the button, and, in about 1 hour, 15 minutes, you have a decarboxylated product. *ardentcannabis.com*

TCHECK
tCheck is an application-specific UV-Vis spectrometer designed to measure the concentration of herbal compounds infused in oils and tinctures. It works by shining a specific wavelength (color) of light through the infusion, and measuring the amount of light that makes it through. This device can be used to determine the potency of your infusions. *tcheck.me*

Bibliography

Atakan, Zerrin. "Cannabis, a Complex Plant: Different Compounds and Different Effects on Individuals." *Therapeutic Advances in Psychopharmacology 2*, no. 6 (December 2012): 241–254. doi:10.1177/2045125312457586.

Bogacki, Olivia. "Vanilla Custard Cookie Cups." Liv for Cake. February 19, 2017. Accessed August 15, 2017. https://livforcake.com/vanilla-custard-cookie-cups/.

Bolognini, D., E. M. Rock, N. L. Cluny, M. G. Cascia, C. L. Limebeer, M. Duncan, C. G. Stott, et. al. "Cannabidiolic Acid Prevents Vomiting in *Suncus murinus* and Nausea-Induced Behaviour in Rats by Enhancing 5-HT1A Receptor Activation." *British Journal of Pharmacology 168*, no. 6 (February 25, 2013): 1456–1470. doi:10.1111/bph.12043.

Butterfield, Delilah. "Cannabidivarin (CBDV): The Cannabis Compound that Treats Epilepsy." Herb. July 30, 2017. Accessed August 15, 2017. http://herb.co/2017/07/30/cannabidivarin-cbdv/.

Butterfield, Delilah. "Marijuana Deaths: How Many are There?" Herb. January 12, 2016. Accessed August 15, 2017. http://herb.co/2016/01/12/many-people-died-overdosing-marijuana/.

CannLabs. "Most Common Cannabinoids." Cannabis Consumer Research. Accessed August 15, 2017. http://cannabisconsumer-research.com/guide-cannabinoids-human-body/.

Cervantes, Jorge. *The Cannabis Encyclopedia: The Definitive Guide to Cultivation & Consumption of Medical Marijuana.* Vancouver, WA: Van Patten, 2015.

ChefSteps. "Pâte de Fruit." Accessed August 15, 2017. http://chefsteps.com/activities/pate-de-fruit.

Christensen, Emma. "How to Make Soft & Chewy Caramel Candies." The Kitchn. November 27, 2015. Accessed August 15, 2017. http://thekitchn.com/how-to-make-soft-chewy-caramel-candies-cooking-lessons-from-the-kitchn-180832.

Demeter. "Paleo Almond Joy." Beaming Baker. September 12, 2016. Accessed August 15, 2017. http://beamingbaker.com/paleo-almond-joy-vegan-gluten-free-dairy-free/.

Fidyt, Klaudyna, Anna Fiedorowicz, Leon Strządała, and Antoni Szumny. "caryophyllene and caryophyllene oxide—Natural Compounds of Anticancer and Analgesic Properties." *Cancer Medicine 5*, no. 10 (October 2016): 3007–3017. doi:10.1002/cam4.816.

Flinn, Melanie. "Coconut Almond Butter Cups." Nutritious Eats. May 27, 2016. Accessed August 15, 2017. http://www.nutritiouse-ats.com/paleo-coconut-almond-butter-cups/.

Floyd, Teresa. "The Fail-Safe Way to Line a Baking Pan with Parchment Paper." Food52. August 14, 2015. Accessed August 15, 2017. https://food52.com/blog/13618-the-fail-safe-way-to-line-a-baking-pan-with-parchment-paper.

Fowler, Damon Lee. "Simple Candied Orange Peel." Epicurious. December 2008. Accessed August 15, 2017. http://epicurious.com/recipes/food/views/simple-candied-orange-peel-350798.

Full Spectrum Labs. "Cannabinoid Cheat Sheet." Cannabis Consumer Research. Accessed August 15, 2017. http://cannabis-consumerresearch.com/guide-cannabinoids-human-body/.

Garten, Ina. "Frozen Key Lime Pie." Food Network. 2002. Accessed August 15, 2017. http://foodnetwork.com/recipes/ina-garten/frozen-key-lime-pie-recipe3-1945602.

Heeger, Susan, and Susie Norris. *Hand-Crafted Candy Bars: From-Scratch, All-Natural, Gloriously Grown-Up Confections.* San Francisco, CA: Chronicle Books, 2013.

Herb. "Decarboxylation: What It Is & Why You Should Decarb Your Weed." November 2015. Accessed August 15, 2017. http://herb.co/decarboxylation/.

Hossack, Izy. "How to Make Dairy-Free Coconut Yogurt." The Kitchn. February 23, 2016. Accessed August 15, 2017. http://thekitchn.com/how-to-make-dairyfree-coconut-yogurt-cooking-lessons-from-the-kitchn-216358.

Hua, Stephanie. "Banana Cream Pie with Chocolate Ganache and Salted Caramel Sauce." Lick My Spoon. December 2, 2010. Accessed August 15, 2017. http://lickmyspoon.com/?s=banana+cream+pie.

Huff, Tessa. "How to Use a Piping Bag." The Kitchn. October 5, 2015. Accessed August 15, 2017. http://thekitchn.com/how-to-use-a-piping-bag-224064.

Kikoko. "Cannabinoid 101." Accessed August 15, 2017. http://kikoko.com/cannabinoid-101/.

Leafly. "Infographic: What are Cannabis Terpenes and How Do They Affect You?" October 14, 2015. Accessed August 15, 2017. http://leafly.com/news/cannabis-101/infographic-what-are-cannabis-terpenes-and-how-do-they-affect-you.

Lo, Monica. "Cuddlenut Oil." Sous Weed. March 16, 2016. Accessed August 15, 2017. http://sousweed.com/blog/2016/3/16 \cuddlenut-oil?rq=coconut%20oil.

Lo, Monica. "Sous Vide Canna Butter." Sous Weed. June 13, 2015. Accessed August 15, 2017. http://sousweed.com/blog/2015/6/13/sous-vide-cannabis-butter.

McDonough, Elise. "Which Fat Absorbs THC Best?" *High Times*. June 1, 2016. Accessed August 15, 2017. http://hightimes.com/edibles/which-fat-absorbs-thc-best/.

McKenney, Sally. "Simply Perfect Vanilla Cupcakes." Sally's Baking Addiction. August 29, 2016. Accessed August 15, 2017. http://sallysbakingaddiction.com/2016/08/29/simply-perfect-vanilla-cupcakes/.

Meadow. "How Is Marijuana Medicine: The Endocannabinoid System." Accessed August 15, 2017. http://getmeadow.com/education/how-is-marijuana-medicine.

Medrich, Alice. *Bittersweet: Recipes and Tales from a Life in Chocolate*. New York, NY: Artisan, 2003.

Michaels, Dan. *Green: A Field Guide to Marijuana*. San Francisco, CA: Chronicle Books, 2015.

Morante, Coco. "Carrot Cake Power Bites." The Kitchn. May 17, 2015. Accessed August 15, 2017. http://thekitchn.com/recipe-carrot-cake-power-bites-snack-recipes-from-the-kitchn-211886.

Muckian, Kyle. "The Big Benefits of Eating Marijuana Rather than Smoking It." Herb. April 28, 2016. Accessed August 15, 2017. http://herb.co/2016/04/28/benefits-eating-marijuana/.

NV Cann Labs. "Get to Know Your Cannabinoids and Their Potential Medical Benefits." Accessed August 15, 2017. http://nvcann.com/science/.

Parks, Stella. "BraveTart: How to Make Your Own Nilla Wafers." Serious Eats. 2012. Accessed August 15, 2017. http://sweets.seriouseats.com/2012/01/bravetart-homemade-nilla-wafers.html.

Parks, Stella. "Macarons." BraveTart. 2011. Accessed August 15, 2017. http://bravetart.com/recipes/macarons.

Prof of Pot. "11-Hydroxy-THC-Increased Potency that Explains the Effect of Edibles?" Accessed August 15, 2017. http://profofpot.com/11-hydroxy-tetrahydrocannabinol-potency-edibles/.

Project CBD. "Terpenes and the 'Entourage Effect.'" Accessed August 15, 2017. http://projectcbd.org/science/terpenes/terpenes-and-entourage-effect.

Ptak, Claire. *The Violet Bakery Cookbook*. Emeryville, CA: Ten Speed Press, 2015.

Rhan, Bailey. "Cannabinoids 101: What Makes Cannabis Medicine?" Leafly. January 22, 2014. Accessed August 15, 2017. http://leafly.com/news/cannabis-101/cannabinoids-101-what-makes-cannabis-medicine.

Rhan, Bailey. "Ingest or Inhale? 5 Differences between Marijuana Edibles and Flowers." Leafly. July 17, 2014. Accessed August 15, 2017. http://leafly.com/news/cannabis-101/ingest-or-inhale-5-differences-between-marijuana-edibles-and-flow.

Rhan, Bailey. "Terpenes: The Flavors of Cannabis Aromatherapy." Leafly. February 12, 2104. Accessed August 15, 2017. http://leafly.com/news/cannabis-101/terpenes-the-flavors-of-cannabis-aromatherapy.

Robinson, Naomi. "Caramel Corn and Pecan Honey Brittle." Bakers Royale. February 7, 2017. Accessed August 15, 2017. http://bakersroyale.com/caramel-corn-and-pecan-honeycomb-brittle/.

Rockwell, Rachel. "Edible Cookie Dough (Microwaved Flour Method)." Sprinkle Some Fun. Accessed August 15, 2017. http://sprinklesomefun.com/2012/04/not-so-raw-cookie-dough-for-eating.html.

Rosenthal, Ed, with David Downs. *Beyond Buds: Marijuana Extract—Hash, Vaping, Dabbing, Edibles, and Medicines*. Piedmont, CA: Quick American Archives, 2014.

SC Labs. "Cannabinoids: The Most Common Cannabinoids Found in Cannabis." Accessed August 15, 2017. http://sclabs.com/cannabinoids/.

SC Labs. "Terpenes." Accessed August 15, 2017. http://sclabs.com/terpenes/.

Shavit, Ori. "Vegan Meringue: The Complete Guide to the Foam that's Taking the World by Storm." Vegans on Top. June 4, 2015. Accessed August 15, 2017. http://vegansontop.co.il/vegan-aquafaba-meringue-english/.

Shinjyo, Noriko, and Vincenzo Di Marzo. "The Effect of Cannabichromene on Adult Neural Stem/Progenitor Cells." *Neurochemistry International* 63, no 5 (November 2013): 432–437. http://doi.org/10.1016/j.neuint.2013.08.002.

Smith, Owen. "The Cannabis-Terpene Synergy." *Cannabis Digest*. March 6, 2015. Accessed August 15, 2017. http://cannabisdigest.ca/cannabis-terpene-synergy/.

Stuckey, Barb. *Taste What You're Missing: The Passionate Eater's Guide to Why Good Food Tastes Good*. New York, NY: Atria Books, 2013.

United Nations Office of Drug and Crime. *World Drug Report 2015*. United Nations. http://unodc.org/documents/wdr2015/World_Drug_Report_2015.pdf.

Wishnia, Steven. "Smoke vs. Snack: Why Edible Marijuana Is Stronger than Smoking." *The Daily Beast*. June 13, 2014. Accessed August 15, 2017. http://thedailybeast.com/smoke-vs-snack-why-edible-marijuana-is-stronger-than-smoking.

World Health Organization. "Information Sheet on Opioid Overdose." Accessed December 17, 2017. http://who.int/substance_abuse/information-sheet/en/.

About the Authors

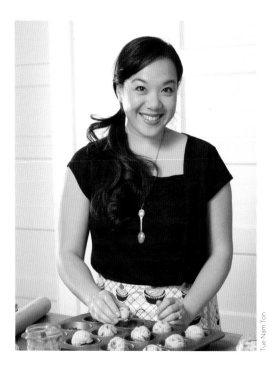

Tue Nam Ton

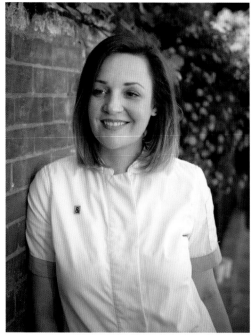

Craig Hackey

STEPHANIE HUA

Stephanie Hua is the founder and chief confectioner behind Mellows, Getmellows.com, gourmet cannabis-infused marshmallows handcrafted in San Francisco, California. Mellows have been featured in the *San Francisco Chronicle, High Times,* and *Dope Magazine,* among other publications. In addition to making edibles, she has been a food writer, recipe developer and tester, and photographer for more than ten years. Stephanie has a culinary arts degree from San Francisco Cooking School and is a graduate of Brown University. Her recipes, writing, and food photography have been featured in *The Huffington Post, Wine Enthusiast Magazine, Fodor's Travel, Serious Eats, PBS, SF Weekly, 7x7,* and KQED's *Bay Area Bites.* She also tested recipes for the James Beard Award—winning cookbook Bar Tartine.

GUILTY PLEASURE MUNCHIES:
Expensive ice cream and cheesy poofs.

COREEN CARROLL

Coreen was born and raised in Germany and moved to Florida in the late 1990s. Having been the oldest granddaughter of a huge family, she spent a lot of time learning kitchen skills and recipes from her mother and grandmother. After getting her degree in International Business at the University of North Florida, she and her now husband moved to San Francisco to follow her lifelong food dreams and achieve a culinary arts degree from San Francisco Cooking School. After working as a butcher's apprentice, she started exploring edible infusions while working in the underground pop-up restaurant world. She cofounded and developed a cannabis edibles company that went on to win multiple awards including Best Edible at the High Times Cannabis Cup San Francisco. Now, she is founder and executive chef of the Cannaisseur Series, Cannaisseurseries.com, which offers an array of curated cannabis dining and pairing experiences in California. In 2017 she was named one of "America's Top 10 Cannabis Chefs" by Greenstate. Coreen and the Cannaisseur Series have been featured by the *San Francisco Chronicle, Business Insider,* Discovery Network, Cannabis Now, and *Dope Magazine,* among others.

GUILTY PLEASURE MUNCHIES:
Cheese, cheese, and, when in doubt, cheese
(and chocolate-covered raisins).

Index

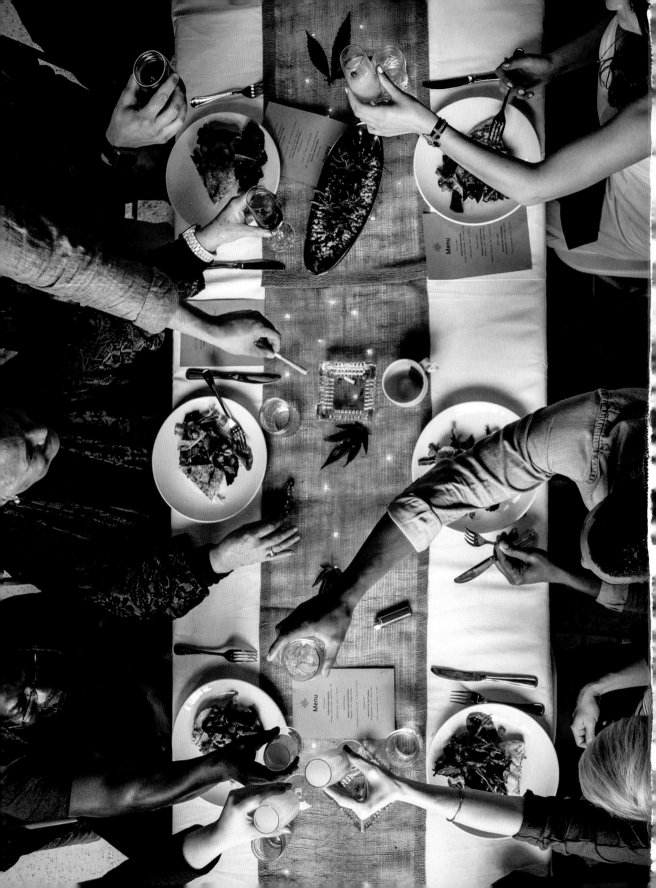

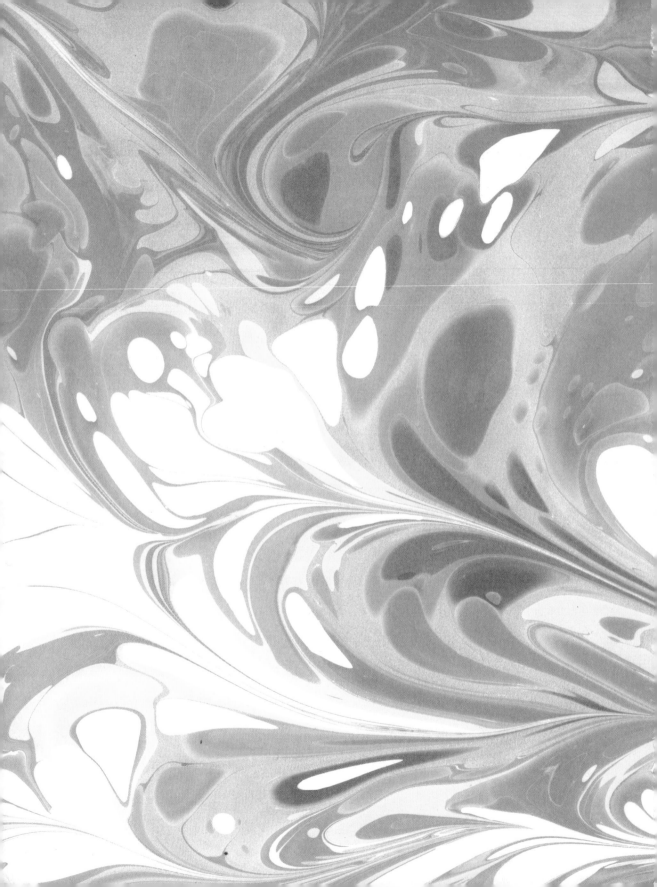